PRAISE FOR *THE BR*

"*The Breath of Life* captures the depth and essen.   ,odynamic craniosacral therapy. Menzam-Sills also includes exerc   .g us into sensation
that ground the work. The book creates a balance be.   concept and fluid based
embodiment of the principles of the work. This is a fantastic book!"

—MARY LOUISE MULLER, RCST®, international teacher, and
cofounder of LifeShapes Institute

"This book is an important contribution to the field of Craniosacral Biodynamics that
beautifully articulates key principles of practice from a feminine perspective. Menzam-
Sills describes the great 'Intelligence' that generates and organises our health and offers
insights from many years of clinical experience, which are interwoven with experiential exercises to provide the reader with an embodied sense of this work."

—MICHAEL KERN, course director of the Craniosacral Therapy
Educational Trust in London and author of *Wisdom in the Body:
The Craniosacral Approach to Essential Health*

"In her new book, Cherionna Menzam-Sills takes us on a journey to understand and
experience Craniosacral Biodynamics. She brings us to the heart of the work with a
personal, experiential approach that deepens and complements her clear expression
of the theoretical basis of Biodynamics. Her style, descriptions, stories and guided
exercises will enliven and enrich understanding for both newcomers and experienced
practitioners."

—ANNA CHITTY, BCST, Biodynamic Craniosacral Therapy
course director, and cofounder of the Colorado School of
Energy Studies

THE BREATH OF LIFE

THE BREATH OF LIFE

AN INTRODUCTION TO CRANIOSACRAL BIODYNAMICS

Cherionna Menzam-Sills, PhD

Foreword by Franklyn Sills

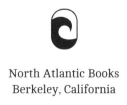

North Atlantic Books
Berkeley, California

Published by
North Atlantic Books
Berkeley, California

Cover design by Nicole Hayward
Interior design by Happenstance Type-O-Rama

Printed in Canada

MEDICAL DISCLAIMER: The following information is intended for general information purposes only. Individuals should always see their health care provider before administering any suggestions made in this book. Any application of the material set forth in the following pages is at the reader's discretion and is his or her sole responsibility.

The Breath of Life: An Introduction to Craniosacral Biodynamics is sponsored and published by the Society for the Study of Native Arts and Sciences (dba North Atlantic Books), an educational nonprofit based in Berkeley, California, that collaborates with partners to develop cross-cultural perspectives, nurture holistic views of art, science, the humanities, and healing, and seed personal and global transformation by publishing work on the relationship of body, spirit, and nature.

North Atlantic Books' publications are available through most bookstores. For further information, visit our website at www.northatlanticbooks.com or call 800-733-3000.

Library of Congress Cataloging-in-Publication Data

Names: Menzam-Sills, Cherionna, 1955- author.
Title: The breath of life : an introduction to craniosacral biodynamics / Cherionna Menzam-Sills.
Description: Berkeley, California : North Atlantic Books, [2018] | Includes bibliographical references and index.
Identifiers: LCCN 2017046680 | ISBN 9781623172053 (trade paper)
Subjects: | MESH: Mind-Body Therapies—methods | Manipulation, Osteopathic—methods | Massage—methods
Classification: LCC RZ401 | NLM WB 880 | DDC 615.8/52—dc23
LC record available at https://lccn.loc.gov/2017046680

1 2 3 4 5 6 7 8 9 MARQUIS 22 21 20 19 18

Printed on recycled paper

North Atlantic Books is committed to the protection of our environment. We partner with FSC® certified printers using soy-based inks and print on recycled paper whenever possible.

*I dedicate this book with
love, gratitude, and appreciation
to my beloved husband,
Franklyn Sills.*

CONTENTS

LIST OF ILLUSTRATIONS

FOREWORD

By Franklyn Sills, RCST

I was so happy when Cherionna decided to write this introductory book on the nature and practice of a biodynamic approach to Craniosacral Therapy. Most of the textbooks in the field have been written by men, yet the vast majority of practitioners are women! It is so important to have a woman's perspective on this wonderful work we do. I am also so appreciative of the style and quality of Cherionna's writing, which I find helps me receive a felt sense of what she is sharing and describing. I also so appreciate the illustrations she created for this book. They again bring a visceral or felt experience into my awareness as I look at many of them along with the accompanying written sections.

I met Cherionna, who is my wife, many years ago at an American Craniosacral Biodynamics conference. She was talking about and demonstrating Continuum Movement, a wonderful movement form that uses movement, breath, sound, and "open attention." Cherionna was an authorized Continuum Movement teacher and was close to her mentor, Emilie Conrad, the founder of the work. Continuum Movement does indeed seem to help participants return to fluidity and ease in their mind-body system and is very resonant with a biodynamic approach. I was so taken by Cherionna's presentation that I approached her after her demonstration, which started us on our lovely interpersonal journey into love, connection, and marriage.

Cherionna is an accredited teacher of Craniosacral Biodynamics in North America and began to assist me in Craniosacral Biodynamics trainings and postgraduate courses, first in the US and then at the Karuna Institute in beautiful Dartmoor National Park in the United Kingdom. Karuna is a residential training center that I helped establish and develop, where we teach trainings and postgraduate courses in Craniosacral Biodynamics, a form of Craniosacral Therapy that we pioneered and continue to develop, which orients us to the formative forces of life. We also teach a mindfulness-based form of psychotherapy, Core Process Psychotherapy, which we have pioneered and developed under the leadership of my former wife, Maura Sills. It has been an incredible journey for me to be involved in these healing arts, and I still appreciate the work that our teachers and students do in their mutual learning processes.

I originally became interested in cranial work in the 1970s when I learned of the work of an osteopath, Randolph Stone. Dr. Stone developed and taught his work from the 1940s through the 1970s. He was a visionary in many ways and perceived the underlying forces and life energies that organize our mind-body system into form. Way back in the late 1940s, he stated that the folding of the embryo at the fourth week after conception into a body form has nothing to do with genes, but with bioelectric exchanges in its fluids. He had interesting images of the fetus organized within energetic fields drawn for his books on Polarity Therapy. However, most osteopaths and doctors around him thought that he was eccentric and deluded. Then, lo and behold, in 2011, modern research discovered that, indeed, the folding of the embryo into a body form has nothing to do with genes, but is a consequence of bioelectric interchange between cells within the fluids of the embryo![1]

I was very taken by Dr. Stone's work with stillness and what he called "the neuter essence," the essence of stillness within all shapes and form, no matter what the conditioned nature of the form is or has become. This led me to attend osteopathic college, where, in an osteopathic apprenticeship, I came across the work of Rollin Becker, DO, and began to orient to what the founder of the work, Dr. William Garner Sutherland, called the "tide," the fluid tide and the stillness at the heart of all form and process. Meanwhile an osteopath named John Upledger began to bring the work out of Osteopathy as "Craniosacral Therapy." Upledger taught a very biomechanical approach to the field, which came out of the earlier work of Sutherland. In his later work, Sutherland emphasized the underlying forces organizing our mind-body system into form, which he called "the potency of the Breath of Life." His work involved much less "doing," with perception of the "unerring potency" and the "tide" of Primary Respiration at its root.

It took my colleagues and me many years to develop an approach to teaching the work in our own context, and it continues to develop and change with every cycle of teaching at the Karuna Institute. The work spread around the world as Biodynamic Craniosacral Therapy as I was asked to teach in many locations, as were many of our senior tutors. Craniosacral Biodynamics has spread in many ways around the world and is a "broad church," with many approaches and many ways of understanding the work. There are biodynamic professional associations around the world, and it is a very exciting time for the work.

What I again feel is missing is the feminine perspective on our work, which is grounded in presence, relationship, and stillness, where the majority of practitioners are female and most of the books have been written by men. So please read and enjoy Cherionna's very visceral and felt journey into a biodynamic approach to Craniosacral Therapy.

Many best wishes, Franklyn Sills

PREFACE

This book began as a seed planted by my husband, Franklyn Sills, pioneer in the field of Craniosacral Biodynamics. He felt there was a need for an introductory text on this beautiful practice. The seed was further watered by conversations with cranial students lamenting the lack of female authors in this field and excited by their experience of Continuum Movement, which I had introduced to them within the context of Craniosacral Biodynamics classes.

During my years with Franklyn, I have undergone dramatic shifts in my own understanding and practice of Craniosacral Biodynamics. I have deepened also in appreciation of Franklyn's ability to articulate the subtle perceptual experiences and healing processes involved in Craniosacral Biodynamics, and to organize them into a coherent conceptual system delivered in a remarkably effective training curriculum. His clarity seemed to dissolve perceptual veils and clouds of confusion for me and many others.

I had been practicing and teaching Craniosacral Biodynamics for some time before Franklyn and I began our personal relationship. Romantic attraction is always a source of ignition and discovery, but for me, our ongoing discussions about the work we share and love further kindled the fire.

I had studied Craniosacral Biodynamics with John and Anna Chitty, who had in turn studied with Franklyn. From working closely with Anna in Boulder, Colorado, while preparing to become a teacher myself, I had shared in her struggles to clarify and develop the work and how to impart it. I loved the energetic field of unconditional love Anna seemed to create in her classes. Although I was already a practicing somatic psychotherapist and specializing in prenatal and birth trauma when I took the Craniosacral Biodynamics training with John and Anna, I found my understanding and ability to work effectively with trauma grew exponentially under their tutelage. I also found my own ability to self-regulate went through a quantum leap while taking their foundation training in Craniosacral Biodynamics.

We all celebrated when Franklyn's first volumes of Biodynamic Craniosacral Therapy were finally published. Until that time, we had available a number of books by cranial osteopaths that related to our work to varying degrees. However, Franklyn's books were actually about what we were doing in the foundation training and could really serve as texts. Teaching this work became a bit easier at that point, but there were numerous discussions between teachers about what it was we were actually doing. There were so many questions.

The two postgraduate seminars I took with Franklyn didn't entirely clear things up for me. They actually sparked more curiosity as I saw that he was exploring areas not covered in his books. When we began to get to know each other, I learned that he considered the original two volumes to be bridge texts, intended to support those trained in more biomechanical forms of cranial work in the transition to a more biodynamic approach. Back in 1992, he and his tutors at Karuna Institute had agreed they weren't teaching what they were actually practicing. They were teaching what Franklyn had believed was necessary to teach to beginning practitioners. They began the process of revising the curriculum to reflect a more biodynamic approach. The trainings he had taught in America and elsewhere had not necessarily reflected this change due to practical issues involved. Much of the confusion we experienced as students and teachers seemed to relate to this discrepancy.

When our personal relationship began, Franklyn was working on a new set of texts relating to how the curriculum and understanding of the work had evolved. I helped edit and review the texts, including contributing my own chapters. I also began assisting Franklyn in his foundation training in New York City. The clouds began to clear! With each *aha!*, I found myself settling deeper into the work. I experienced my perception clarifying in astonishing ways, which continues even as I write this. I am also witness to Franklyn's ongoing development, as he further elucidates and simplifies aspects of the work. I feel deeply grateful for the opportunity I have had to be so close to Franklyn and his evolving clarity in this field.

As I continue my own journey with biodynamic practice, I enjoy bringing my own touch (yes, feminine touch) to the work. My other passion is Continuum Movement, founded by my mentor, the late Emilie Conrad. Continuum is a mindful movement practice profoundly feminine in many ways. It is all about curves and spirals, pulsations and waves. Like Craniosacral Biodynamics, it involves slowing down and deepening into fluid, spacious states accompanied by subtle perception. It utilizes different breaths, vocalized sound usually directed into the body tissues, body movement, and subtle awareness. I consider it an embodied mindfulness practice, potentially altering the nervous system and enhancing a sense of health, wholeness, and well-being.

An inspiring Continuum teacher Bonnie Gintis is also a Biodynamic cranial osteopath. In her book, *Engaging the Movement of Life*, she compares the two practices.

She writes, referring to founder William Sutherland, founder of Cranial Osteopathy, "Sutherland considered the goal of Osteopathic treatment to be the free movement of all the fluids of the body across their interfaces. Continuum practice addresses the same issues by empowering each individual to engage their own fluidity and to stimulate movement of the fluids themselves as well as the body as the fluid container."[2] In Craniosacral Biodynamics, we particularly orient to the organizational forces affecting the free or inhibited flow within the body. In Continuum, we can sense and embody these subtle influences. I have heard many declare that Continuum is like giving yourself a Craniosacral or Biodynamics session.

It was actually through my presentation on Continuum and Craniosacral Biodynamics at a Biodynamic Craniosacral Breath of Life conference in North Carolina that Franklyn and I began our romantic relationship. I had originally called the presentation "Continuum and Biodynamics: A Perfect Marriage." I later changed the subtitle to "Parallel Paths," but was reminded by biodynamic colleagues of the original title two years later when Franklyn and I married.

When I was encouraged by a male student to write this book because of lack of female voices in this field, I realized it would need to include a Continuum influence. I can no longer practice Craniosacral Biodynamics without referring to Continuum. Throughout this book, I offer guided experiential, body-centered explorations primarily influenced by Continuum.

My take on Craniosacral Biodynamics is often visual as well as somatic. I literally see Craniosacral Biodynamics in beautiful luminescent images. It challenges my artistic and digital skills to attempt to portray what I see on these pages, but I delight in the challenge and hope you do, too!

This book is, in a sense, an expression of the marriage of my two loves! I hope it will provide for you the kind of igniting spark I have received in discussing Craniosacral Biodynamics with Franklyn, and that I continue to receive in each treatment session.

I offer in the following pages insights from my own journey, as I have sought to clarify and embody the principles and concepts of Craniosacral Biodynamics. I welcome you to this evolving and dynamic field, which, as you will see, is about our most essential being.

my life. I so appreciate the Chittys' teaching, which led me into teaching Craniosacral Biodynamics. Anna in particular demonstrated for me a feminine, heart-centered approach to teaching that I wanted to emulate.

I also want to acknowledge and appreciate the support of my biodynamic colleagues, other biodynamic tutors and trainees, too many to name individually here, who applauded and encouraged me along the way. This includes a special thanks to Michael Kern for his generously offered editorial feedback and to Katherine Ukleja who joined me in exploring the feminine in this beautiful work. The book changed character in response to comments of the tutor team at our training in New York City who told me that not only they but also their clients were eagerly awaiting my book. I realized then that I could include clients and potential clients in the audience for this book.

I also want to include the teachers I have had along the way who encouraged me in my writing, artwork, and somatic exploration. I cannot omit from this list my beloved mentor, the late Emilie Conrad, founder of Continuum. This mindful movement form influences everything I do and is between, if not in, every line of this book. Emilie also encouraged my writing. She used to say to me, "If you ever can't do cranial work, you can always write!" Thank you, Em. I am now writing!

I gratefully thank my editors and the publishing staff at North Atlantic Books for so warmly welcoming and expertly guiding the birth of this book.

Finally, I thank my friends and others who have patiently waited for me to be more available socially and who have offered feedback and encouraged me in this creative endeavor. Thank you to all who had faith in my ability to bring forth a book worth reading. May it bring you deeper health, peace, and well-being.

1
Beginnings:

Overview and Brief History of Craniosacral Biodynamics

*S*tanding *beside the treatment table, where my client lies comfortably, I feel my heart soften and expand as I remember the sacredness of the journey we are embarking on together. I have already guided the client in orienting to a sense of resource. She has recalled a favorite big tree she often visits. Taking a deep breath, she has reported a sense of her own roots into the earth and an ability to rest into them, standing tall like the tree she identifies as her resource. I have suggested she take this image and felt sense to the table with her, where I have guided her in being aware of her breath and the places where her physical body makes contact with the table, sensing the support of gravity under her body.*

I explain I am settling myself further in relationship to her, as I stand at the side of the table. Within my own system, I orient to my own sense of contact with the support of the earth through my feet, my own breath, my own body. I begin to settle deeper into a sense of the wholeness of my body, and its fluid nature, as I allow my awareness to soften and widen. I sense fields within fields of support holding me and my client as I widen my attention and allow the client's midline to become the center of my perceptual field. There is an almost palpable sense of softening and settling in the space between us as our relational field settles.

Again, I am reminded of the sacredness of our journey. I rest in gratitude for the opportunity to be able to practice and share this biodynamic presence with another…

And so, you and I begin our biodynamic journey together in this book. My intention is, as in session work, to guide you in your ability to rest into the support of universal forces, to orient to the profound and seemingly limitless intelligence of what we call the Breath of Life and its tidal expression as Primary Respiration. We begin with a look at the historical context and evolution of this powerful work of Craniosacral Biodynamics.

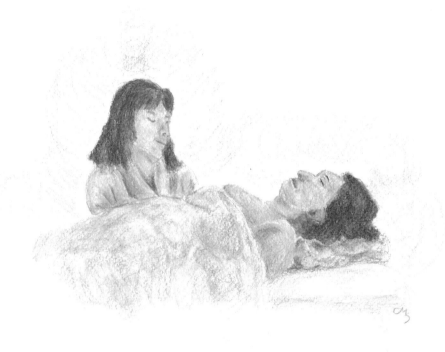

FIGURE 1: Biodynamic Craniosacral Therapy Session

Craniosacral Biodynamics is a gentle, sensitive form of a hands-on approach to health that has evolved from the work of the early American osteopath, William Garner Sutherland, and other osteopaths following in his footsteps, such as his student, Rollin Becker. More recently, within the context of Craniosacral Therapy, Franklyn Sills has also pioneered in this field, particularly through further clarification of essential concepts and processes, and through developing a coherent, dynamically evolving curriculum to teach it outside of the context of Osteopathy. The essence of Craniosacral Biodynamics is an orientation to deep formative forces of life, rather than just the effects of these forces, such as morphology (shaping), tissue organization, and symptoms. As Sills states, "The intention in this work is to learn to relate to the forces present in patterns of distress in the human system, not just to the resultant and compensatory tissue and fluid patterns or inertia."[3]

The term *biodynamic,* as used by Sills, was borrowed from osteopath Rollin Becker, who in the 1960s described "biodynamic intrinsic forces" and "biokinetic" externally derived forces.[4] It is important to understand this historical source, as there are other forms of bodywork and cranial therapy also using the term *biodynamic* with different sources and different meanings. Please understand that my intention here and throughout this book is to clarify what is meant by the term in the approach developed by Franklyn Sills, with all due respect to practitioners with alternative orientations to Biodynamic work.

When I mention to people that I practice Craniosacral Biodynamics, they sometimes assume this relates to the Biodynamic Psychotherapy developed by Gerda Boyesen or the work of Rudolf Steiner, who established a form of agriculture called biodynamic farming. I am not an expert on Steiner's philosophy, but my understanding is that biodynamic farming, like Craniosacral Biodynamics, is a very holistic approach. Farmers consider phases of the moon to determine when to plant or harvest crops. Biodynamic farms aim to grow food within a natural, balanced environment, where birds, animals, and all kinds of plants are equally welcomed, as are elemental beings and fairies. Steiner espoused a deeply spiritual, heart-centered approach to life. As I have heard his followers point out, this has parallels to the philosophy of Craniosacral Biodynamics.

A contemporary of Steiner and Sutherland was Erich Blechschmidt, a German embryologist who also used the terms *biodynamic* and *biokinetic*.[5] Because Craniosacral Biodynamics involves perception of the universal forces that underlie our early formation in the womb, as well as throughout our lives, some practitioners associate the terms with Blechschmidt's work. Blechschmidt, however, was interested in morphology, defined as "the branch of Biology that deals with the form of living organisms, and with relationships between their structures."[6] In other words, he described the dynamic changes in the shape and structures of the embryo. Craniosacral Biodynamics, as taught by Sills, utilizes perception of the forces responsible for that morphological development. While they are related, they are not identical. Morphology arises as an effect of underlying formative forces. These include both universal biodynamic forces and biokinetic forces related to an individual's conditions in life. The Craniosacral Biodynamics we discuss in this book involves sensing and working with the underlying forces influencing embryological and later formation. Our intention is to observe the effects of these forces from the inside of the individual, rather than trying to change the form from the outside. The purpose in learning about embryological development from this perspective relates to understanding the forces involved in our formation, both as embryos and throughout life.

Craniosacral Biodynamics is based on perceptual experience. The forefathers preceding us, like current teachers in the field, attempted to put their perceptual experience into words, to guide others along a similar path. Here I am reminded of stories I have encountered of Buddha's attempts to pass on his wisdom. When followers begged the awakened one to enlighten them, he would describe the path available to them. He could guide them to the path, but it was up to them to walk it. Similarly, we attempt to clarify a path for students of Craniosacral Biodynamics to develop their skills, but each must learn through practice. One of the influences Sills brought to this work was his experience as a Buddhist monk. Before discussing more fully Sills's contributions, however, I would like to describe some of the foundational inquiry from which Craniosacral Biodynamics has grown.

Early Pioneers

The ground of Craniosacral Biodynamics was laid by early osteopaths. Andrew Taylor Still, father of Osteopathy, explored the ease of movement of bones and other structures in the body. He did not include the cranium as the cranial bones were believed to be immobile, a common belief in America and much of the West, but not held in Italy and more eastern locations.[7] Still did, however, value the cerebrospinal fluid bathing the brain and spinal cord. He stated:

> A thought strikes him that the cerebro-spinal fluid is one of the highest known elements that are contained in the body, and unless the brain furnishes the fluid in abundance, a disabled condition of the body will remain. He who is able to reason will see that this great river of life must be tapped and the withering field irrigated at once, or the harvest of health be forever lost.[8]

William Garner Sutherland, a student of Still, became curious about the cranial bones, leading him to become father of Cranial Osteopathy (also known as Osteopathy in the cranial field). Sutherland's initial work was inspired by an unusual thought occurring to him while viewing the temporal bones of a disarticulated skull. He wrote, "The thought came to me 'beveled like the gills of a fish and indicating a *primary respiratory mechanism,*' not only struck me, it stayed with me. That was how I came to undertake a study intending to prove to myself that mobility between the cranial bones in the adult is impossible."[9] Figure 2 compares the beveled edge of the temporal bone with the gills of a fish. How does this visual affect you? Do you sense a resonance between the two?

Given that the beveled edge of the temporal bone suggested that the joint between it and its neighboring cranial bone was designed for movement, Sutherland began exploring ways to restrict the hypothesized cranial bone motion to prove it wasn't

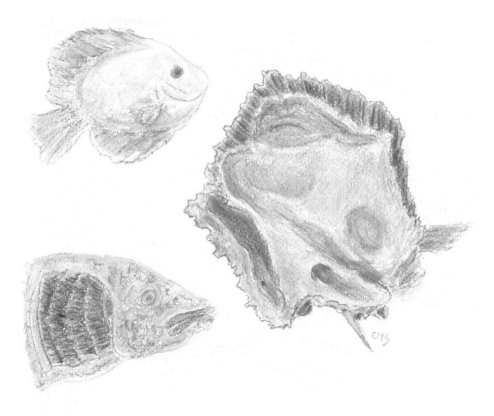

FIGURE 2: Beveled Like the Gills of a Fish

happening. Expecting no results from bracing his skull with rubber bands, kitchen bowls, leather straps, football gloves, etc., he discovered, much to his wife, Adah's, dismay, that his brain and nervous system function were impaired by his experiments. He then developed ways of remedying the damage through using his hands on his own skull.[10]

Sutherland studied and practiced for about forty years, over which time his perception and understanding evolved from focusing on movement of the bones to gradually include in his "Primary Respiratory Mechanism" meningeal membranes in and around the brain; cerebrospinal fluid within and around the brain and spinal cord; cranial-pelvic connections; and the brain and nervous system. His Primary Respiratory Mechanism included five important areas:[11]

1. Inherent fluctuation of cerebrospinal fluid

2. Motility of the neural tube (central nervous system, or CNS)

3. Reciprocal tension membrane (the dural meninges surrounding the CNS)

4. Articular mobility of the cranial bones

5. Involuntary motion of the sacrum between the ilia

These continue to be important in many forms of cranial therapy. Over the years, Sutherland's cranial concept became increasingly holistic and subtle. He began to speak of the Breath of Life and Primary Respiration, differentiated from the breath of air or secondary respiration of the lungs. He wrote, "According to biblical history: A breath of LIFE was breathed into the nasals, and man became a *living soul.* Note that it was a breath of LIFE, not the breath of *air;* the breath of *air* being one of the material elements that the breath of LIFE utilizes in a mechanism to walk about upon earth."[12]

Sutherland perceived a process of "transmutation" of what he termed the Breath of Life. Transmutation refers to a changing of state or stepping down into increasingly dense, physical expression. For example, in figure 4, we can see the formation of the heart as energetic forces organized by the Breath of Life spiral and coalesce, guiding the cells and tissues into this physical form.

Sutherland saw this Breath of Life as a mysterious, larger source beyond the physical body. He sensed through his "thinking-feeling-seeing-knowing fingers" the subtle,

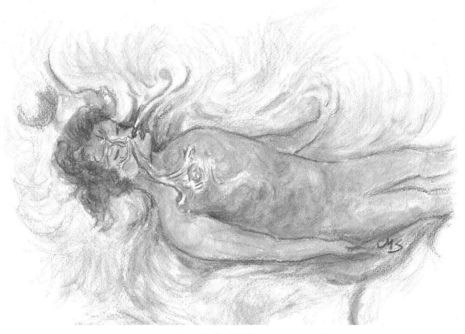

FIGURE 3: Breath of Life Blown into Nostrils

rhythmic fluctuations of fluid within the body. He perceived the cerebrospinal fluid (CSF) in the ventricles of the brain picking up the "potency," or life energy, of the Breath of Life, the fountain of this force that forms us. The CSF then carries this potency to every tissue, every cell in our bodies, bringing life and health.[13]

The five areas of anatomy comprising the Primary Respiratory Mechanism then become less important. Rather, the underlying breathing of Primary Respiration in every cell becomes of interest. The sacrum may be moving in relation to the ilia on either side of it (mobility), but all the bones, as well as the connective tissues between

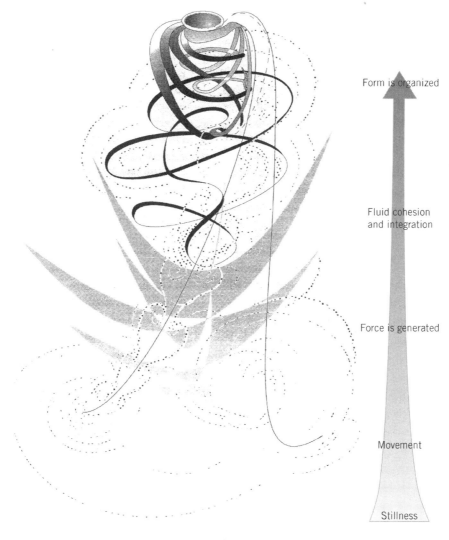

Form is organized

Fluid cohesion and integration

Force is generated

Movement

Stillness

FIGURE 4: Transmutation
Illustrator Dominique DeGranges, in Sills, 2001, Figure 7.2, p. 103

them and the cells forming them, are filling and emptying together, as one unified field of motion, with each inhalation and exhalation of what has come to be known as the mid-tide. This inherent motion of every cell and tissue of the body with Primary Respiration is known as *motility*. This contrasts with *mobility*, which refers to the motion of parts in relation to each other. Sutherland's initial study of the movement of the cranial bones involved their mobility. This was a natural focus of perception emerging from his training as an osteopath to orient to the motion or immobility of bones. As his perception became more subtle and holistic, he recognized the deeper, more intrinsic motion of motility, indicated by the arrows in figure 5.

Toward the end of his life, Sutherland had a direct experience of the Breath of Life at the bedside of a dying man, surrounded by his family. Sensing a healing force moving through the man from beyond the physical body was a profound experience that altered Sutherland's way of working. While most forms of Craniosacral Therapy are based on Sutherland's earlier work, Craniosacral Biodynamics evolves from this later phase of Sutherland's discoveries.

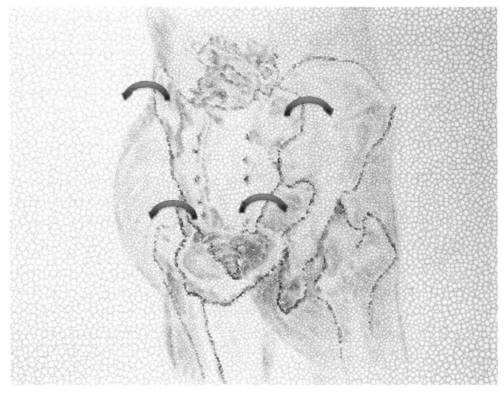

FIGURE 5: Cellular Sacrum Breathing

His work in this final decade of his life was characterized by less active doing, and more attention to deeper forces. He advised his students to "rely upon the Tide." He wrote:

> Visualize a potency, an intelligent potency, that is more intelligent than your own human mentality ... You will have observed its potency and also its Intelligence, spelled with a capital I. It is something you can depend upon to do the work for you. In other words, don't try to drive the mechanism through any external force. Rely upon the Tide.[14]

The meaning of this advice has taken time for cranial practitioners to integrate. As interpreted by some, relying upon the tide is a highly foreign approach in the modern Western world. It involves a major paradigm shift. This was as challenging for osteopaths in Sutherland's day as it is for many practitioners and students now. Sutherland's discussion of the ephemeral Breath of Life was not well received. Many osteopaths rejected Sutherland's later explorations, continuing with the more physically based practices he had developed previously.

Earlier in his career, Sutherland had practiced various forms of subtle manipulation of cranial bones, membranes, ligaments, and fluids. Most cranial practitioners today continue to practice such manipulations. These "biomechanical" techniques involve the common cultural perception of the body as a living machine. When something goes wrong with a machine, the mechanic evaluates what is wrong, which informs how to fix it. When I broke my wrist recently, for example, it was extremely helpful to have an X-ray taken so as to establish which bones were affected and if they were truly broken. Then a skilled practitioner could set the bone and immobilize it with a cast. This is a useful, biomechanical approach. It involves the external source, the X-ray technician, the doctor, etc., evaluating the situation and applying an external force, X-rays and a cast, to fix the problem.

An example of a biomechanical approach in Craniosacral Therapy is depicted in figure 6. Here the therapist is evaluating a torsion pattern in the cranial base (occiput, temporal, and sphenoid bones) by subtly encouraging the torsion motion with their hands, as indicated by the arrows.

Craniosacral Biodynamics is a different approach, evolving from Sutherland's later teachings. It involves appreciation and facilitation of the deeper formative forces, as well as their often less subtle effects. Different from biomechanical approaches, our orientation is primarily to these underlying forces, rather than their effects, including the symptoms clients may present. For example, in figure 7, you can see a force spiraling into what we call an organizing inertial fulcrum within the spheno-basilar junction

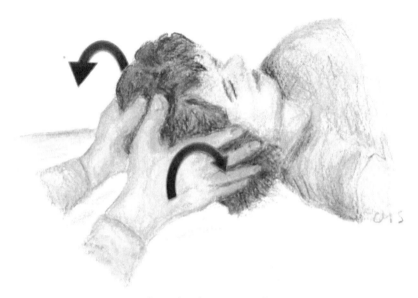

FIGURE 6: Biomechanical Evaluation Cranial Base Torsion Pattern

(the joint between the sphenoid bone and the base of the occipital bone). A fulcrum is a point of stillness, which has an organizing influence on the tissues. (See chapter 5 on the inherent treatment plan for a fuller explanation.) In this case, the movement of these bones of the cranial base is limited on the right side by the inertial pull of the fulcrum. The inertial pattern in the tissues may be sensed throughout the cranium and even reflected lower in the body. The practitioner holds in awareness this fulcrum within the whole field, rather than manipulating the tissues to find the pattern and compressive effects resulting from this fulcrum.

Continuing my personal example, in a previous fall, I injured my other wrist. While I was grateful to receive biodynamic sessions to support the healing, I found it important to have an X-ray and an MRI to determine that the bones were bruised rather than broken. I also happily wore the splint provided to aid the bones in recovering from their assault. I valued these biomechanical interventions as much as the biodynamic sessions. Craniosacral Biodynamics, however, augmented my body's natural healing abilities, and accelerated and eased the healing process, along with my own movement meditation practices. I am reminded that there is a time and a place for everything!

Rollin Becker

One of Sutherland's students, Rollin Becker, espoused Sutherland's later explorations and continued to develop and articulate the dynamics of Primary Respiration. As

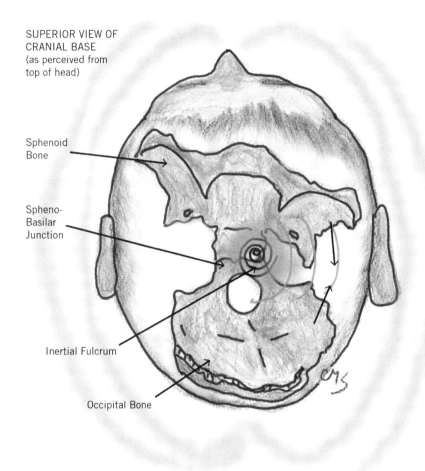

SUPERIOR VIEW OF
CRANIAL BASE
(as perceived from
top of head)

Sphenoid
Bone

Spheno-
Basilar
Junction

Inertial Fulcrum

Occipital Bone

FIGURE 7: Biodynamic Holding of Inertial Fulcrum

mentioned earlier, Becker coined the term *biodynamic,* to refer to intrinsic, universal forces influencing our body formation throughout life.[15] He differentiated between biodynamic and *biokinetic* forces, which relate to our individual conditions caused by external forces. These biokinetic, or conditional, forces can include exposure to toxic substances or drugs, the impact of accidents, injuries, surgeries, and other external conditions. Even our genetic makeup can be considered biokinetic. At any given time, we are under the influence of both biodynamic and biokinetic forces.

Biodynamic forces resemble, and perhaps are, the universal embryological forces that form us in the womb. Becker writes, "The bioenergy of wellness is the most powerful force in the world. It is dynamic. It is rhythmic. It is a force field that begins with the moment of conception and continues to the last moment of death."[16]

Early in our development, all embryos resemble each other. Our earliest development, as we shall see, is directed by universal energetic forces, rather than by genes that determine our individual differences. All embryos take shape in relation to an energetic midline. The work of scientist Mae-Wan Ho demonstrates that even microscopic

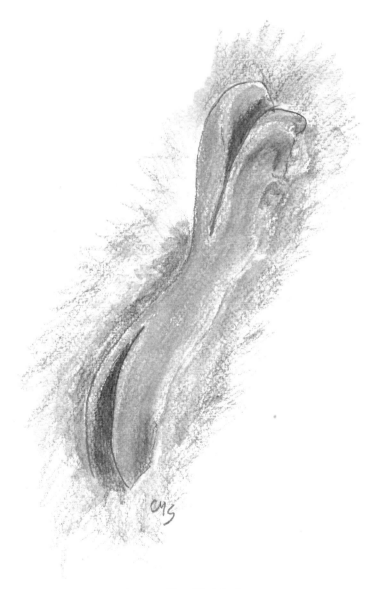

FIGURE 8: Three-Week Embryo

creatures have an energetic midline responsive to their environment and apparently organizing their form.[17] A group of scientists recently studying frog embryos observed a bioelectric interchange between cells as the form of the embryo's face formed energetically before it took form physically. You can view this fascinating development on YouTube, where an energetic midline also appears to present before the midline develops physically.[18] It seems that an energetic field is established at conception, providing guidance for the embryo's formation.[19] Supporting this understanding of an energetic ignition, a flash of light has been observed by researchers using fluorescent indicators at the moment of conception during in vitro fertilization.[20] Significantly, the stronger the flash, the more likely was the embryo to survive. We apparently depend on this mysterious bioenergetic force for our formation and survival.

This phenomenon expresses truly universal principles of creation. We can see the same principles at work in formation of stars in the cosmos as we see in the embryo. In each case, a field is established with a still point as fulcrum in the center. Rhythmical expansion and contraction in relation to this fulcrum, like a universal breath, underlie formation. For example, figure 9 depicts a spiral galaxy with its central point of light *Notice how your body and breath respond as you gaze upon this beautiful image from the Hubble telescope. Can you sense a similar spiraling in and out within your own energetic field?*

Craniosacral Biodynamics involves attention to such subtle energetic phenomena, rhythmically re-enacting the miraculous expression of the life force through embryological development. We attend to the subtle motions referred to as Primary Respiration, a subtle breathlike phenomenon that precedes the "Secondary Respiration" starting at birth. These are expressed as what we call the tides.

The life energy driving this expression is essential to health. Sutherland termed this energy "potency."[21] We recognize that potency, as a primary ordering force, is always present in the system, although it may be tied up in areas of holding or compression in the body-mind, or the body and mind as one continuous unit. These "inertial fulcrums" are actually expressions of ever-present health. The system has done its best to manage unresolved traumatic forces by containing them in various patterns in the body-mind. That health is always present is one of the foundational principles of Osteopathy as defined by A. T. Still. He taught osteopaths to orient to health rather than disease, writing, "To find Health should be the object of the physician. Anyone can find disease."[22] From this osteopathic perspective, Becker wrote:

> We have heard for years that the body has within itself all the factors with which to maintain health and to heal itself in case of disease or trauma. This statement is basically true.

The body has the capacity to express health through this inherent potency, and it has the capacity to maintain compensatory mechanisms in response to trauma or disease through variant potencies. At the very core of total health, there is a potency within the human body manifesting its interrelationship with the body in trauma or disease.[23]

Our job as practitioners includes perceiving and resonating with the potency and health in the client, supporting them in resolving issues and expressing more fully. Sutherland referred to an intrinsic "Intelligence, spelled with a capital I" guiding the treatment.[24] The client's Intelligence knows what it needs to do, what needs to be addressed when. As Becker noted, it has its own "inherent treatment program."[25] Biodynamic practitioners

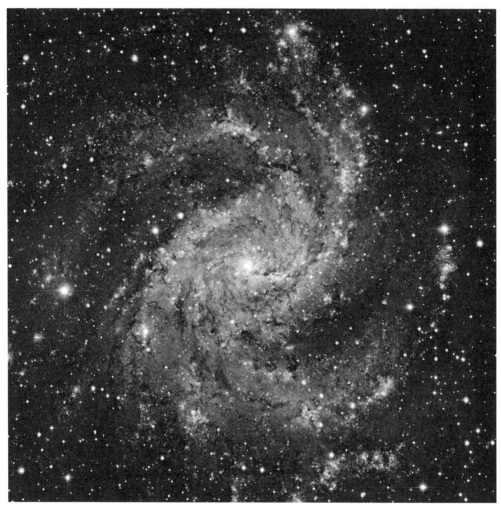

FIGURE 9: Spiral Galaxy
NGC 6946 (HST, Subaru), http://hubblesite.org/image/3678/gallery.
Credit: NASA, ESA, STScI, R. Gendler, and the Subaru Telescope (NAOJ)

have profound respect for this expression of Intelligence. We patiently wait for it to unfold, rather than imposing our own ideas of what should or shouldn't happen or be treated next. This is a most humble practice!

Sutherland had advised his students to "be still and know."[26] As his work became more subtle and less physical, he appreciated more fully the inherent intelligence of the client's system in healing. Becker further instructed his students to do nothing until they experienced a shift to wholeness and Primary Respiration.[27] Where many practitioners would consider this state the end of treatment, Becker saw it as the beginning. It was only when the client's system could settle under all its activity that it could express its inherent treatment program. Sills has extrapolated on this perceptual experience, what he terms the "holistic shift," describing detailed steps often experienced as what he terms the "inherent treatment plan" unfolds.[28] This will be described more fully in chapter 5.

Settling, Softening, Deepening

In order for what we call the inherent treatment plan to present itself, there is usually a need for the client's system to slow down. It is common when we first make contact with a client's body to sense rapid pulsations of an activated nervous system. We often sense fluctuations and wave motions pulling our attention in various directions. Where there is trauma or holding in the system, there is the tendency to focus in on that issue. This limits access to the resources of the entire system.

As practitioners, we settle ourselves before and during work with clients so we can provide a calming, grounding presence for the client's system to resonate with, to remind it of its inherent health and support it in orienting with us to Primary Respiration—"Be still and know." Our intention is to hold an awareness of the patterns and issues presenting within the whole, from a wider orientation to the deeper formative forces establishing and maintaining them. We listen for expressions of the Breath of Life as subtle tidal, or breathlike, motions of Primary Respiration. Over time, usually, the system settles under the waves, fluctuations, and pulsations. Something deeper emerges. Often there is a deep breath as the system begins to feel more whole and fluid. From this place, the intelligence of the system begins to express more clearly. We will review this process in detail in chapter 5.

Franklyn Sills

Franklyn Sills studied at the College of Osteopaths in London, where he was fortunate to intern with an osteopath who had studied with Becker. While working in this office, Sills was exposed to these less popular concepts in Cranial Osteopathy. Later, through his busy practice in London, he further developed his skills. When requested by an osteopathic colleague to develop a curriculum for teaching these skills outside of osteopathic college, Sills incorporated other techniques he had acquired along the way. He had come to Osteopathy via Polarity Therapy, and had already developed and taught a Polarity Therapy training. This work of Randolph Stone had introduced him to energetic healing and orientation to an energetic midline.

As mentioned earlier, Sills had also spent time as a Buddhist monk. In addition, he had studied tai chi and chi kung with very advanced teachers in California. He found the mindfulness presence of these practices helpful for students and practitioners in settling with a client, dropping into a more receptive state where subtle energetic phenomena could be perceived and supported. Sills also drew on his experience with prenatal and birth therapy with William Emerson and Core Process Psychotherapy (CPP). He helped develop and still teaches CPP, which was founded by his previous wife, Maura Sills. These therapies influenced the curriculum Sills developed to include a strong emphasis on establishing a safe relational field. The work included supporting clients in practicing mindful presence and orienting to what helped them through their process. At a conference in the late 1990s, Sills met Peter Levine, founder of Somatic Experiencing (SE), who suggested that their work had clear resonances. This meeting, along with his CPP background, influenced Sills to incorporate an explicit understanding of emotional processes and central nervous system activation into the biodynamic practitioner training. These included various trauma skills and more specific ways of accessing a felt sense of resource and wellness.

As well as these relational components, some other contributions Sills has made to cranial therapy depart from traditional cranial osteopathic and Craniosacral Therapy approaches and techniques. For example, attending to what was called balanced ligamentous or membranous tension shifted to orienting to a deeper state of balance of the forces generating the tension in the tissues. Within the field of Craniosacral Therapy, made popular by John Upledger, Sills heightened awareness of Sutherland and Becker's work among nonosteopathic practitioners of healing arts. He introduced an understanding of the inherent treatment plan, the natural unfolding of healing processes within the expression of Primary Respiration. As mentioned earlier, Sills also included terms like *holistic shift*, relating to Becker's admonition to not do anything before perceiving a shift to wholeness and Primary Respiration as a starting point for the whole session.

More recently, Sills has expanded on Sutherland's later tendency toward nonaction. Interaction with tissue patterns has progressed from relatively active biomechanical manipulations, to more subtle conversational skills, such as suggesting or inviting space within tissue relationships, to more recently practicing augmentation of the life forces, or potency within the space. This shift involves doing less and orienting more to what is already naturally present or arising. For example, rather than actively disengaging compacted sutures, the practitioner, using conversation skills, might ask the tissues if they would consider taking more space. Recognizing that even a subtle invitation was application of an external force, which could have undesirable repercussions, Sills moved on to an even less active intention of augmentation, applied only when the system seems unable to resolve a particularly stagnant issue. Augmentation involves perceiving the natural increase in potency and relationship to space within all tissues occurring in inhalation of the Primary Respiration, and allowing the hands to subtly breathe a bit more with this inhalation quality. Here, a subtle shift in practitioner orientation can support the client's system in also orienting to the potency and space available.

Supporting this less active way of being with a client's system, Sills has also recently introduced into his trainings, starting with the first module, a practice inspired by his chi kung experience. He calls it "Three Body Chi Kung." The practitioner stands by the side of the treatment table before making physical contact with the client and settles into a sense of a three-body suspensory system: physical body suspended within a more holistic fluid body (related to a slow, rhythmical mid-tide expression of Primary Respiration), suspended within a very large tidal body (related to the very slow, long tide). More on this follows in chapter 4.

A Biodynamic Journey

In Craniosacral Biodynamics, as developed by Sills, we gently develop our relationship and physical contact with our clients with an intention to enhance their sense of safety and trust. We support them in being present with their breath and bodily sensations, to balance the tendency to slip into old trauma-related patterns of dissociation or acceleration. We help them to orient to the "resources" available to them. The term *resource,* similar to that used in the Somatic Experiencing work developed by Peter Levine, refers to anything that helps us to stay present, to manage and be with our experience. This may include pleasant, grounding, or even just "OK" body sensations. *What feels OK in your body just now as you are reading this page?* Other resources include things that are working well in the client's life, people or pets they love, activities they enjoy, etc. We track these as the client's system settles and balances.

At some point, we experience a holistic shift. Here, the client's system shifts its orientation from its presenting patterns and conditions to wholeness and Primary Respiration. The system's accelerated, often chaotic, state settles into holistic coherence. This is much like how water in a bottle settles after it has been shaken.

Consider that our bodies are made up mostly of fluid. At our rapid speed of modern Western life, these fluids can be in a state of perpetual shaking. Our nervous systems are constantly in defensive fight-flight or freeze, which interferes with our innate ability to rest, rejuvenate, and relate socially to others in present time. In Craniosacral Biodynamics, we wait for the system to settle before bringing attention to specific issues in the body. Once this settling has occurred, potency naturally begins to orient itself to where it is needed. The inherent treatment plan can emerge when the system no longer needs to constantly respond to external input. As practitioners, we listen for what the client's system chooses to express and follow its lead.

Listening in this way can be compared to going to the woods with the intention to observe wild animals there. If we go thrashing about through the forest, looking for a fox or deer, we are less likely to be rewarded than if we sit quietly and wait. When we are quiet, the animals feel safe to peek out and see who we are. If we continue to be quiet, they come right up to us and curiously start sniffing. If we remain quiet and respectful of their presence, they may then go about their business and allow us to learn from them.

Fluids behave the same way. They show their true nature to us when we quietly witness. If we try to intervene, they react to our actions and intentions. Even such a subtle intervention as looking directly at an animal can alter its behavior. In biomechanical approaches, more focused viewing is helpful in making a diagnosis. In Craniosacral Biodynamics, we need to relearn how to perceive in a more diffuse way, taking in the whole, as little children do, rather than focusing narrowly on an issue. When we receive the issue as part of, even suspended in and supported by, the whole, it can more easily access the resources available to it within the whole.

We can understand this process in terms of quantum physics. In the quantum world, everything exists with potential to be expressed in different ways. Consider the well-known slit experiment, where a single photon (packet of light) passes through two slits as a wave, at times being perceived as a wave and at other times as a particle. Its presentation as one or the other seems to be available as a probability, affected by how the experimenters' attention is directed. Indeed, "quantum phenomena seem to be called into existence by the very questions we ask nature, existing until then in an undefined fuzzy state."[29] In Craniosacral Biodynamics, it is as if we orient more to the wave than to the particle, supporting the benefits of wavelike or tidal manifestation. This is a broader, more inclusive expression than occurs in particle orientation. As we melt into the more fluid, expansive wave state, a sense of more coherent wholeness emerges. Every change is reflected within the whole system. This is different from orienting primarily to the particulars presenting within the whole, such as how one bone moves in relation to another, which is more useful in a biomechanical approach.

While the subtle manipulations of biomechanical work can produce immediate results, they are often followed by efforts of the client's system to integrate the changes that have been externally initiated. Allowing the changes to emerge from internally generated forces enables the whole system to adapt as it needs to. The changes are integrated as they happen, when the system is ready for them.

In some ways, this approach is much easier on the practitioner. We don't need to strive, claim, or pretend to know what is needed. We also don't get to claim responsibility. The work is done by the Breath of Life as it operates through both client and practitioner. There is a resonance between us, which is a key to how Craniosacral Biodynamics works. Simply speaking, we can say that, as fluid beings, the water in me as practitioner communicates with that in the client. We know that water is a highly resonant element. It has been shown to respond to words and intentions.[30] As my system settles and becomes calmer, it reminds the client's system of what it is capable. As the client's system settles and becomes more fluid, mine does too. We say, "Give a session, receive a session." I have never felt burned out doing this work. Even if I have been wearing myself out in my life, I feel better after facilitating a biodynamic session.

For our egos, this approach may be challenging. The little ego self wants to be in control, to be appreciated, to be important. Every time I facilitate a session, I sense my little ego self having to let go. I consider this work to be a form of spiritual practice. My original Biodynamic Craniosacral teacher, Anna Chitty, notes that we are meditating in relationship.[31] As we sit in the presence of another human being, we practice calming our minds and observing our breath and bodily sensations. Often, we enter into a profoundly peaceful state of presence, together with the person on the table. While the little ego self may struggle to be in charge, it also has the opportunity to rest and experience how it is held within the larger field from which we emerge. The mysterious source that forms us, the Breath of Life, rocks us gently in her cradle. As we sit with our clients, it becomes more and more difficult to deny the power and support of this Breath.

Over time, we settle more and more deeply into the rhythms of the Primary Respiration, slowing down until we know ourselves as something deeper, slower, smoother, softer, wider than our everyday personalities. We find ourselves becoming one with the stillness that is us, that is beyond us. We sense ourselves returning, together with our client, to the beginning, prior to the hurts and traumas of our personal histories. Like the early embryo, we float within the full potential of what life has to offer. This is the heart of Craniosacral Biodynamics.

An Experiential Inquiry into the Energetic Nature of Our Bodies

It is not unusual to experience the body as a solid, physical structure. This is, after all, what we were all taught in school, if not before. We cannot walk through walls, and it can hurt to try. At the same time, we live in a world where the mind of science is shifting. While we have all learned about the rules of gravity and how to operate in a Newtonian state, we have also been exposed to revolutionary declarations from the world of quantum physics assessing all things as being aspects of one continuous whole. As David Bohm wrote, "Relativity and quantum theory agree, in that they both imply the need to look on the world as an undivided whole, in which all parts of the universe, including the observer and his instruments, merge and unite in one totality. In this totality, the atomistic form of insight is a simplification and an abstraction, valid only in some limited context."[32]

We seem to be beings of light and space, rather than the solid forms we tend to see and feel. For example, cell biologist Bruce Lipton points out that we can only see each other because light photons bounce off the energy of the otherwise invisible human body.[33] Apparently, our bodies compose themselves from used stardust that has arrived on earth after stars have died or galaxies exploded.[34]

Clearly, there is some mystery involved in our bodies in that they appear physical but consist of energy and light. Rather than attempting to further explain this phenomenon, which we directly perceive in Craniosacral Biodynamics, I would like to guide you in a brief exploration of this matter (pardon the pun) through your own body experience. If you are curious, please settle yourself in a comfortable position and let's begin the journey! You may want to record these instructions in your own voice to enable you to explore with your eyes closed, if you find that helpful, but this is not necessary. You can also listen to a recording of me reading the instructions (available at www.birthingyourlife.org/the-breath-of-life-book).

Take some time to get comfortable in your seat. Notice what sensations inform you in this process. Now, let yourself include one hand in your awareness. Take a moment to squeeze and open this hand three or four times, really letting yourself feel the muscles working and the tissues contracting and expanding. What are those sensations like? Does it feel hard or soft? Warm or cool? Tight or loose? Tense or relaxed? (See figure 10 below.)

Now, slow down the movement. Let yourself orient more to the sensations involved in moving than in the end goal of making a fist or opening your hand. As you slow the movement down, how do your sensations change? Do you sense them only in your hand, or do you sense anything being affected elsewhere in your body? You may begin to have more of a sense of flow, of ease, of fluid wholeness, where more of your body is involved. There may be a sense of energy elsewhere in your body, or perhaps a wave moving from your hand up your arm and through your chest. Your head and neck may begin to want to move, or even your feet. Let yourself be curious, slowing the movement down more and more. (See figure 11 below.)

After a few minutes of exploring this more fluid state, let the movement slow down even more, so it becomes more about stillness than movement. Let your focus be more on the space

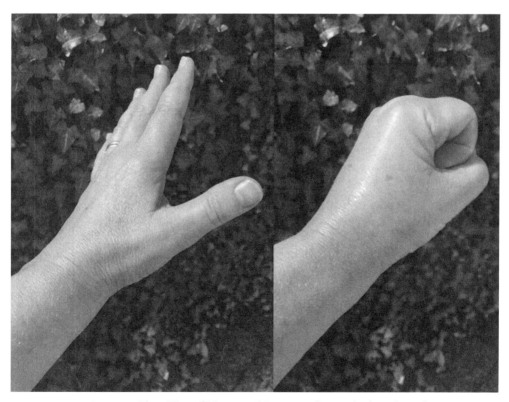

FIGURE 10: Three Ways of Moving and Perceiving the Hand: Physical Hands

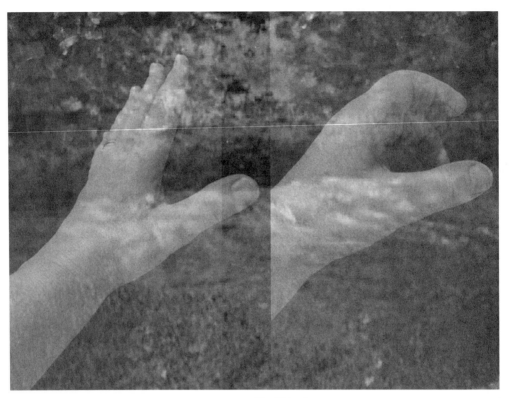

FIGURE 11: Fluid Hands

between your fingers and around your hand than on the micromovements of the hand, itself. What are the sensations like now? It is not unusual in this slow state, with a wider field of orientation, to begin to feel like your hand is not so physical. It may begin to feel more like energy, suspended within a larger field of energy. Notice how it is for you (see Figure 12, p. 23, cosmic hands). When you feel done with the process, or no longer interested, come back to the sensation of your physical hand and body, and look around to orient yourself.

Chances are, if you explore this repeatedly, you will find yourself experiencing increasingly slower movement, with an enhanced energetic awareness. If you stay with this, you may even begin to find some familiar aches and pains dissolving, as a kind of inherent treatment plan spontaneously emerges and healing ensues. We have entered now the mysterious realm of Craniosacral Biodynamics! Welcome!

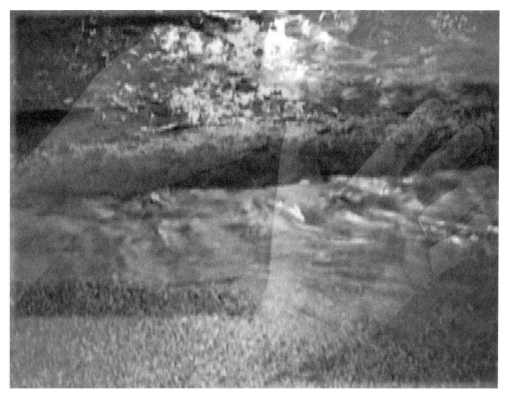

FIGURE 12: Cosmic Hands

2
Practicing Presence

Find your place and close your eyes
so your heart can start to see
...your being will become a great community
—RUMI

We can consider our presence as practitioners to be the first step in our biodynamic journey. We cannot come into relationship with our clients without being present. Our aware presence with clients creates a safe relational field, offering a different context from the one in which trauma and wounding may have occurred earlier in life. Within this field, the client's system and tissues can begin to settle under their historical wounding patterns. As the practitioner holding presence within this relational field orients to the deeper universal forces of Primary Respiration, the client's system is facilitated in deepening further through resonance. Practitioner presence is therefore an important element of the work, supporting both the client's system in settling and the practitioner's ability to sense subtle expressions of the client's physical and emotional history and health.

Practicing presence is not unique to Craniosacral Biodynamics, but it is so essential I have decided to devote an entire chapter to this topic. Presence is essentially one's ability to be aware in current time, which includes being attentive in relationship with others, such as with clients. This chapter discusses the importance of presence in the healing relationship in Craniosacral Biodynamics and offers guidance in deepening your ability to be present with yourself, your body, and whomever you are with. We discuss recent scientific research supporting the practice of mindful presence with oneself and in relationship, and explore how these can affect the inherent treatment plan in Craniosacral Biodynamics.

Let us begin by exploring presence as an expression of and a gateway to being, a natural state of existence where nothing is required of us. In the next chapter, we will discuss the importance for little ones (babies and children as well as the little one consciousness of clients) of being able to rest within a safe relational field where, as pediatrician and psychotherapist Donald Winnicott noted, they can "simply be."[35] In this state, the child, or client, is free to develop according to their natural inherent intelligence. We naturally arrive and grow in a state of being, which Winnicott differentiates from reacting to challenges in our environment.[36] Where this state has been impeded by lack of safety or resonant relationship, the individual develops reactive, defensive ego structures and behaviors. These states are reflected as tensions and holding within the physical body. When we as practitioners try to meet our clients within this influence of our own personal histories, we may easily misperceive what is being presented to us, projecting our own needs and stories onto the client. We will discuss this in more detail later. For now, it is important to note that our emphasis on presence is designed to facilitate deepening under our own history, as well as that of the client, enabling a true, resonant meeting of two beings. It is within this field of presence that healing and our original potential naturally arise.

Presence, like being, has a non-doing aspect to it. If we are simply present, we don't have to *do* anything. There is a sense of stillness and aliveness. It is possible to be present while being active, but this usually takes practice. For example, how aware are you in this moment of your breath as you are reading?

Presence, Breath, and Being

In this section, we practice simple breath awareness and how it can affect our ability to be with ourselves and with others. If we are alive, we are breathing. This means that breath is always available to be aware of. Meditation classes often begin with breath awareness exercises. For most of us, this requires sitting quietly. Once we are accustomed to noticing the breath, we can more easily do it while active. In the beginning, we need to practice in a relatively quiet setting until we develop the neural pathways involved in sensing the subtler sensations of breathing.

Take a moment now to sit quietly and observe your breath. Just let yourself be aware of what you are aware of when you have the intention to be with your breath. Can you sense the breath? If so, where in your body do you sense it? What qualities do you notice in the breath? How fast or slow is it? How easy or effortful? How deep or shallow?

When we first begin attending to our breath, we often find it is fast and shallow. This reflects the state of the nervous system. Most of us in our modern Western world spend much of our time under the influence of an activated sympathetic nervous system. This aspect of the autonomic nervous system prepares us for fight or flight, and enables our alertness during the day. In support of being able to fight our foes or flee from them, the sympathetic nervous system accelerates our breathing and directs blood away from the organs of digestion and reproduction and toward the more immediately necessary heart, lungs and big muscles of the arms, legs, and jaws. Our breath accelerates and we tend to pant, rather than breathing more deeply into the belly.

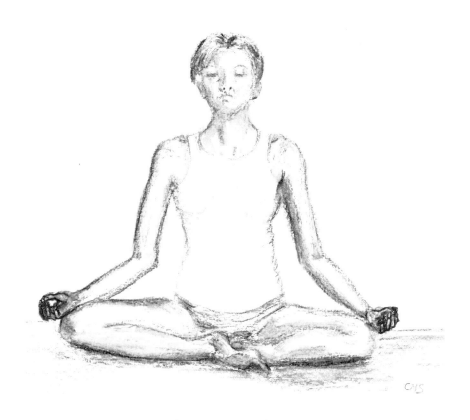

FIGURE 13: Practicing Presence

As we sit and begin to relax, usually our breath becomes slower and fuller, moving the belly, as the parasympathetic, or rest and rejuvenation, nervous system becomes more active and blood is again directed to the organs in the belly. (A recording of this exploration is available at www.birthingyourlife.org/the-breath-of-life-book/.)

Take a moment now to notice your breath again. How fast or slow is it now? Where do you sense it? Do you feel it in your nostrils? In your chest? In your stomach/diaphragm area? This isn't about trying to make your breath any particular way, just noticing how it actually is. Does it go down into your belly? You may want to support your ability to sense the movement of the breath by putting one hand on your chest and one on your belly. Do they move with each breath in and out? Perhaps one moves more than the other? You may sense all of your breath in your chest area, or all in your belly.

I have noticed with the increasing popularity of yoga and other kinds of body-work and relaxation techniques a tendency for people to breathe in their bellies because they have been taught to do so. Our lungs, however, are above our bellies. As they fill and empty, the chest is designed to expand and contract. The rib cage and its associated connective tissues stretch and relax along with the diaphragm. When we limit the movement of the breath to the belly, the tissues of the upper trunk, including those around the heart, can become rigid, leading to health problems, as well as limiting the breath. On the other hand, it is not unusual for people in perpetual fight-or-flight mode to breathe primarily in the chest, with limited movement of the diaphragm curtailing the fullness of the breath.

Some of us hardly breathe at all. *How is your breath now? Have you been able to find it when asked?* I would guess at least some readers find their breath too subtle to sense. This is nothing to be worried about or ashamed of. It is simply your starting point, how it is in this moment, and has the potential to change over time.

Being aware of the breath is a basic aspect of mindfulness practices, derived from the teachings of the Buddha. Buddha discovered through his own practice that simply observing the reality as it is, without trying to change or control it, practicing being aware and equanimous (equally being with and accepting of all situations), leads to liberation from human suffering. As you practice being aware of your breath, your mind may wander. Mindfulness meditation includes being aware of when you lose your focus, acknowledging your mind's meandering, and gently returning to your breath, or whatever you were focusing on. Being kind or friendly toward yourself and your experience supports your learning, as well as your sense of equanimity. Recent research demonstrates that this kind of awareness practice changes our neurobiology, as well as our sense of well-being.[37]

Parts of the brain involved in present-time awareness develop as we practice attending to current experience. This requires practice because most of us spend much of our time not in present time. Buddhist teacher Tara Brach notes that whenever we hear ourselves saying "should," as in "I should be different," it is a sign that we are not being present with what is, because we are needing it to be different.[38] How often do you feel or say that word *should*?

When we experience fear, it is similarly not about this moment. It relates to what *could* happen in the future based on our experience in the past. It is important to be able to predict the effects of our actions, which involves projecting into the future. It is important to be able to learn from the past. Most of us, however, suffer because we become stuck in the past or are already living in the future. *Have you ever had an embarrassing moment that you couldn't stop replaying in your mind? Or have you ever been anxious about an upcoming event and spent the whole night unable to sleep because you were preparing for it in your head? As you remember these events, what happens to your breath? How is your breath in this moment? Does anything change within you as you come back to your breath?*

When we are fearfully reviewing the past or anxiously anticipating the future, our defensive nervous systems are activated. The amygdala, a small almond-shaped part of the brain, serves as a sentry. Always on the lookout for danger, it evaluates our current level of threat based on past experience. If incoming stimuli resemble past danger in some way, the amygdala alerts us to potential hazard. Our sympathetic fight-or-flight nervous system is activated. We are alert, ready to defend ourselves when the danger presents. *Notice how reading this affects your breath.* When you bring your attention to your breath, a different part of the brain, the prefrontal cortex, is activated. This more recently evolved part of the brain is involved in present-time awareness. It also is an aspect of the social engagement nervous system, a concept proposed by neuropsychiatrist Stephen Porges.

In the 1990s, Porges revolutionized psychotherapy and trauma therapy by introducing his Polyvagal Theory.[39] You probably learned in school about the sympathetic and parasympathetic nervous systems, and how they must be in balance for good health. The sympathetic fight-or-flight system relates to the sympathetic chain of nerve centers running down each side of the spine. The parasympathetic rest and rejuvenation system relates to the vagus nerve, a cranial nerve supplying various organs. *Vagus* means "wanderer" and the vagus is the longest nerve in the body, with many branches wandering to and from the different organs in the trunk. Porges realized that the vagus nerve was actually more than one nerve, emerging from different nuclei, or nerve centers, in the brain stem. (Hence the term *polyvagal,* meaning "many vagal.") The old vagus, normally associated with the parasympathetic system, arises from the dorsal nucleus. The new vagus, both new to our knowledge and more recently evolved, arises from the nucleus ambiguus, and is closely associated with several other brain nuclei (nerve centers in the brain) responsible for facial expression, speech, and the senses involved with our social interactions. Porges termed this the social engagement system. He noted that in evolutionary terms, this is the most recently developed system.

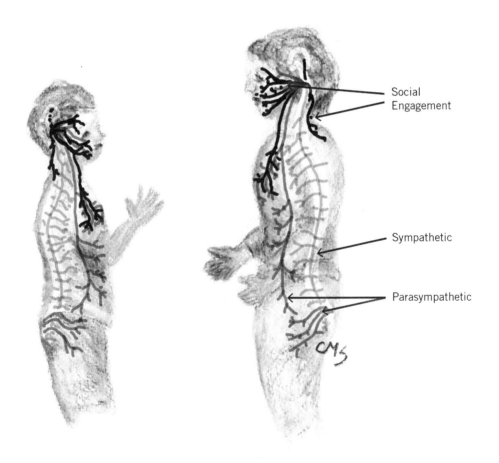

FIGURE 14: Polyvagal Nervous System

Relatively simple organisms early in evolution had parasympatheticlike responses, being able to withdraw, immobilize, and reduce oxygen intake when in danger. Sympathetic functions, involving mobilization, evolved later, with legs in vertebrates supporting the ability to mobilize. The social engagement system developed in mammals, where the young require extended periods of parenting until mature enough to function more independently. The social engagement system, particularly developed in primates, supports bonding and attachment, and protection of offspring.

For humans, who are physically relatively weak, small animals, the social engagement system has supported communal, cooperative living. We have safety in numbers. We can protect each other and use our cooperative skills and language to build protective shelter and tools. Porges noted that, when faced with potential threat, our nervous system responds hierarchically, relating to when each system developed in evolution. Our first response to threat as humans is to use our social nervous system to look toward other humans. We check to see if anyone else is nearby and how others are responding to the suspicious sound, movement, etc. If we are with others, we communicate about our experience and, together, find ways to deal with it. As primates, this is our first impulse when threatened or stressed. If this most recently evolved nervous system response doesn't work, we go to the defensive system that evolved before it—the sympathetic. If that doesn't work, our parasympathetic freeze response sets in.

The parasympathetic nervous system not only slows us down when we are able to rest and recover from a sympathetic surge needed for survival in a threatening situation, but it also enables us to freeze or "play dead" when our sympathetic system isn't adequate to protect us. If a saber-toothed tiger approaches, we evaluate whether we are capable of fighting or need to run away. If neither option works or is possible, we then enter a parasympathetic immobilization or freeze state. Designed to lessen our pain if we are eaten or to make us less appealing to predators who are hopefully less attracted to dead meat, this extreme parasympathetic reaction enables us to dissociate, deadening our senses. We become numb, as well as paralyzed.

We can easily see this in babies. When something stresses them, they begin with a social cry or sound. It has the feeling of, "Hey, Mom, I need you. Please come." If Mom doesn't respond, the baby's cry eventually changes. It begins to sound angry and demanding as the sympathetic nervous system is activated. *Mom! Where are you! Come now!"* If Mom still doesn't come, the baby eventually stops crying, becoming still and quiet. In nature, this may be an adaptive mechanism, as a quiet baby is less likely to be noticed by a predator. Unfortunately, this parasympathetic dissociative response is often misread in babies. The baby is considered a "good baby" who doesn't cry, doesn't create a bother, and doesn't make demands. If you look at such a baby closely, however, you see the eyes have a faraway, vacant look. In a craniosacral session, when you are holding a baby or client in such a dissociative state, it feels like no one is home. There is a sense of deadness, numbness, or emptiness.

We will look further at this kind of response in clients in chapter 7, which discusses working with trauma. For now, it is helpful to understand that unresolved trauma in our system can affect our ability to be present and to sense our breath and body sensations. This can be the effect of an activated sympathetic state, where we are oriented to danger and tend to perceive it everywhere. It can also relate to a habitual parasympathetic dissociative state, where we tend to be numb, not sensing current sensory stimuli. Porges points out that the social engagement system can come back online when we settle these defensive reactive states.[40] Our perception literally shifts as the social engagement system enables us to accurately perceive social relational cues and to recognize safety when it exists. We then come back into relationship in present time. We become capable of immobilizing without fear, resting in relational safety.

Presence, Heart, and Being

Breath awareness is a simple way to begin coming back into present time. *Are you aware of your breath just now? Take a moment to come back to breath or deepen into this awareness again.* Including the heart in our awareness can quickly reawaken the social engagement system. The new vagus nerve supplies the heart and lungs, conducting important messages from the heart to the brain, as well as from brain to heart. Breath and heart function are closely related. *While you are being with your breath, can you also feel your heartbeat? To facilitate this, I suggest putting one hand over your heart. What do you sense? How is it to have your hand on your heart? Can you feel your hand touching your chest? Can you feel your chest from your hand? Can you feel your hand from your chest? Take a little time now to listen to your heart. Can you feel it beating? How fast or slow does it beat? How hard or soft is the beating? It may feel very subtle or it may feel like your heart is pounding out of your chest. Or somewhere in between.*

I find the work of the HeartMath Institute extremely helpful in deepening into presence, particularly in relation to the heart. Since the 1980s, HeartMath has focused on researching the intelligence and physiology of the heart and how to access it for meeting life stresses more easily and successfully. The HeartMath research demonstrates that heart awareness affects heart function, which in turn regulates physiology, emotions, and behavior, enabling more coherent, resilient, and functional responses to stress and life. Just being aware of the heart can have a calming, regulating effect. HeartMath technologies include simple methods for sensing the heartbeat and measuring heart rate variability (HRV), the beat-to-beat changes in heart rate found to be associated with health and resilience, and the ability to adapt one's behavior as needed to meet current conditions. HeartMath research has also shown a relationship between HRV and a state of coherent or harmonious resonance between the body's oscillatory systems and between individuals. Everything in our bodies, as in all nature, is vibrating and subtly breathing. We shall explore this more in chapter 4 in relation to the subtle rhythms we perceive in Craniosacral Biodynamics.

Every organ in the body has its own rhythm, as well as moving subtly with what we call the tides of Primary Respiration in Craniosacral Biodynamics. In our modern

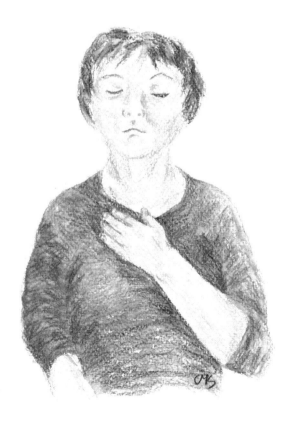

FIGURE 15: Sensing the Heart

Western world, we tend to think of the brain as being in charge of our bodies and behavior, but the research shows that the heart is in fact the leader. The bioelectric field of the heart is sixty times larger than that of the brain, while its biomagnetic field is even greater—5,000 times that of the brain.[41] These fields apparently carry information between individuals, as well as within one's body. In that Craniosacral Biodynamics primarily works through energetic resonance augmented through the practitioner's system, the heart fields may be particularly important in this work. We often practice resting in our hearts as we hold a client, allowing our presence to emanate from the heart.

As mentioned earlier, the vagus nerve carries messages between heart and brain. It turns out there are many more neural pathways going from the heart to the brain than the other way around. The heart-to-brain messages provide important information for self-regulation. The heart is a sensory organ. Its messages are essential to health and well-being. We all know it is important to "listen to our hearts," but how often do we actually

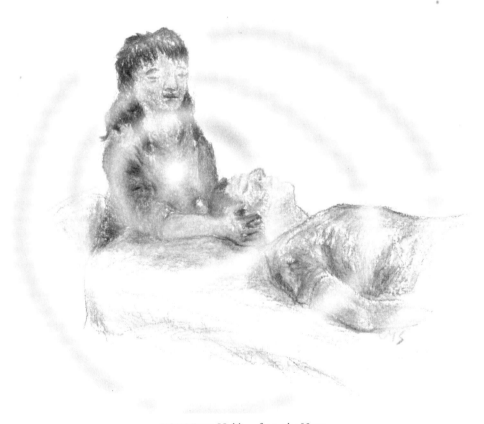

FIGURE 16: Holding from the Heart

do so? *Take a moment now to listen to your heart. Put your hand over your heart again and listen or sense. What are you aware of? Does it feel different than it did earlier? Can you sense the heart beating now? Is it easier to sense now or is it more elusive?* As we become quieter, the heartbeat softens, but with practice, our awareness also becomes subtler.

If you stay with this exploration long enough, you are likely to find the heartbeat coming more into focus. Similarly, if you focus on your breath, it will tend to present itself more clearly. *Can you sense it now? Has it changed at all?* I suggest taking a break from reading here to sit for at least ten to twenty minutes with your breath and your heart. If you can't sense both at the same time, don't worry. Take some time to be with your breath; then shift your attention to your heart. Then you can return to your breath and continue this way for the full time. You may find yourself being more interested in either the breath or the heart. Take note of your preference, and spend some time with the one you prefer. Then to expand your repertoire, take some time to be with the other. This is about equanimity, rather than reinforcing your habitual preferences. It is about *being* with, rather than trying to *do* anything.

You began breathing the moment you were born. And your heart has been beating since four weeks after you were conceived! At that time, you were not as active as you are now. You were floating in fluid within your mother, doing nothing, simply being. Taking this time to be with your heart and your breath can help you return to that original state of being. As a little embryo, just being and growing, your senses began to develop long before you were born. In the next section, we will explore how to awaken sensory awareness beyond the heart and breath.

Presence, Sensation, and Awareness

Mr. Duffy lived a short distance from his body.

—JAMES JOYCE, *Dubliners*

How present are you with the sensations of your body resting on the chair or whatever you are sitting on? Even the simple act of reading can distract us from simply being with our own bodies. The question then becomes, if I am not with my body, where am I?

Most of us in the modern Western world, like James Joyce's character, Mr. Duffy, live disconnected from our bodies. We learn when we are little to dissociate from our bodies. I remember when I was six or seven years old being required to sit at my desk in school with my hands clasped in front of me with an upright "perfect" posture. I think this was supposed to make us into good children with good learning habits (like "good" babies who don't cry or make a fuss because they are dissociated; these babies are not quite there). I now know how difficult it is for a young child to take in and process information without movement. We learn through our bodies. Children with learning difficulties often benefit immensely from practicing developmental movements like going back to crawling on the floor, which helps the nervous system rewire and integrate in a way that may have been missed earlier.

There are many possible events inhibiting or reducing movement in children, which can in turn inhibit or interfere with learning. For example, when I treat babies, their parents sometimes bring them to me in a car seat. They explain that the baby was sleeping and it was easier than waking them up. I always cringe in these situations. Not only is carrying a car seat much harder on the parent's body than holding a baby close to the body, but also the baby is missing out on important movement and kinesthetic stimuli and synchronization through being in a linear boxlike car seat. Babies carried close to the body receive the sensory stimuli of the curves of the parent's body to mold into, with all its interesting variations. The parent's body provides warmth, a heartbeat and breath to resonate with, as well as the sounds of the heartbeat and the voice nearby. A car seat just isn't the same! Staying in the car seat also means the child misses out on reaching out to the parent, sensing the parent's hands and arms making contact, adjusting to the changes in relationship to gravity, etc. An occasional experience in a car seat isn't going to be harmful for most children, and the speed and complexity of modern life may demand this, but being carried around this way repeatedly certainly has an influence. If the child has had previous or additional events supporting dissociation, the car seat can serve to reinforce the tendency, rather than providing opportunities for healing. Sitting still in school may just be adding insult to injury.

Unfortunately, for some of us, like me when I was a child, sitting still and being good weren't that difficult. I had already dissociated from my body years before. My mother had been given general anesthesia during my birth. This affected both of us, rendering neither of us being very present for the event. As a result, I was pulled out with forceps, depriving both my mother and me of the natural dance of birth, the rhythmical coordinated pushing of little baby feet against the toned uterine wall as it contracts. Perhaps in part because of this, I was what would today be called developmentally delayed. I never crawled and didn't walk until I was almost two years old. Having missed out on being present with each other at birth, it was fifty years before my mother and I actually bonded! This happened through movement, when we were dancing together, for the first time in my life, at a family reunion. Our hearts resonated and our social engagement systems awakened as we gazed into each other's eyes, like moms and babies do just after birth. (You see, healing can happen at any time! There is always hope, always potential as health is always present and seeking expression.)

Babies are designed to be alert and mobile at birth. At the first birth I attended, the baby lifted her head and looked around the room, making eye contact with each person present, almost before her whole body had been born. Bonding is a form of learning. We look deeply into each other's eyes and hearts, learning about each other and our relationship. If we are cut off from our sensations, as when anesthetized or in a traumatic freeze state, we have difficulty moving. If we are separated from our body movement, for example by being forced to sit still in school—or standing or sitting in a corner as punishment, or being strapped in a stroller instead of being worn by Mom—we have trouble sensing. When faced with an intolerable experience and unable to escape by running away (sympathetic nervous system), we shut down (parasympathetic immobilization). When punished instead of soothed for being emotional or upset, we learn to not feel the emotions or upset.

Like many other children, by the time I was seven, I had learned to ignore the important messages from my body sensations and instead to listen to my intellect. Other traumatic events in my childhood reinforced the dissociative tendencies established at birth with the anesthesia. Re-embodying involved years of mindfulness meditation, bodywork, somatic psychotherapy, and work with my prenatal and birth experience. It is because the fruits of these practices have been so delicious that I teach and write about these things. I can't imagine how I would be able to be with my clients or sense the subtle phenomena we do in Craniosacral Biodynamics without having done this work on myself. I know that learning Craniosacral Biodynamics was immensely facilitated by years of Vipassana meditation, which both taught me to be aware of breath and body sensations, and to be able to be present with the subtle aliveness to be found in stillness. (Vipassana, derived from the teachings of the Buddha, involves observing breath and bodily sensations, practicing awareness and equanimity—being nonjudgmental without preference for whatever arises.)

Finding Sensations in the Body

We have already begun exploring awareness of sensations through focusing on the breath and sensing the heart. You would not be aware of the breath if you did not feel the sensations of the breath moving in and out of your body. You may feel the touch of the breath in your nostrils or just below them, above the upper lip. Or you might sense the movement of your chest, stomach, belly, or other parts of your body with the breath. I invite you to take a little time now to explore this. *Sit comfortably in a quiet place and close your eyes, if you are comfortable doing so. Otherwise, you can keep your eyes open with a soft focus. The intention is to reduce external distractions and enhance your awareness of your breath and body. Let yourself become aware of your breath again. As you do so, become curious about the sensations that inform you about the qualities of your breath and where it moves in your body. If, for example, you find your breath to be rapid and effortful, how do you sense this? Do you sense the breath moving in your nose? Do you sense the movement of your chest? As you are with the breath for a while, you may find it slowing down. Where do you sense this? What sensations tell you the breath has slowed? You may find you become aware of more movement in your belly where previously it was primarily in your chest. Can you feel the sensations of that movement?*

One way to become aware of sensation is through noticing the places the body makes contact with the surface it is on. As you are sitting, can you feel your seat? Can you feel the weight of your body resting into the chair? Or do you have a sense of pulling up away from the chair? You may even have a sense of floating above the chair. You can also explore this lying down. Lying on your back provides many more places of contact to detect. You may want to read this over first and then lie down and observe, or you may want to record yourself reading these guiding questions and listen to them when you are lying down. (A recording is available at www.birthingyourlife .org/the-breath-of-life-book.)

Can you sense your body as you shift your position into lying down? Once you are lying on your back, explore the contact in different parts of your back. Check your upper back, middle back, lower back. There is a natural arch behind the neck and lower back. How big is this arch? Can you put a hand through the space between your lower back and the floor/ mat/bed you are lying on? This suggests an emphasized arch, suggesting this part of your body is pulled up away from the support of gravity. Do you feel tension here?

I like to think of Mother Earth as always there under us, holding us in her lap. To what extent do we allow ourselves to yield into that support? Where do you sense your body yielding or resting into the support of gravity? Can you feel the weight of your body sinking into the floor? Are your shoulders touching the floor? Or are they lifted up and away from it? Are they both the same? Are there differences between the right and left sides of your body? Again, this isn't about trying to make things any particular way, but about just being aware of how they actually are in this moment. How about your upper arms? Can you feel them? Elbows? Forearms? Wrists? Hands? Are your hips and pelvis resting into gravity? What is the contact with the earth like there? Can you feel their weight into the earth? Check the backs of your legs and feet.

Being with the back of your body also offers a different perspective on the breath. When you breathe, your contact with the floor shifts slightly with each breath. As you breathe in, your body volume increases slightly. There is a slight increase of pressure into the floor. As you breathe out, the body volume decreases slightly and the pressure into the floor slightly lessens. Can you feel this? Take your time. Allow yourself to be with these sensations. Allow yourself to be curious. What can you feel? What can't you feel? Does it change as you are with it for a while or if you come back to it later? If you aren't feeling much, take note of that. Is it possible to be curious about your lack of awareness? What might have contributed to it? Is it possible to have compassion for yourself if you are not sensing what you think you should be? This is just how it is in this moment. It will change, as all things change.

A traditional mindfulness meditation is to sit quietly, being aware of your breath, and then to begin expanding your awareness to include more of your body. You can literally scan your body from head to toe, checking what your sensory awareness is like in each place. Alternatively, you can begin with your breath, gradually including more parts of your body. In my Continuum classes, I guide people through sensing their breath in the usual places—nose, chest, diaphragm, belly—and then point out that the breath is designed to carry oxygen and life to every cell in the body and to take carbon dioxide and other wastes away from every cell. It is possible to sense the breath everywhere in the body. *Can you sense it below your belly, down into your pelvis? Your hips? Your thighs? Knees? Lower legs? Ankles? Feet? Every cell in your body is breathing. Can you feel them? Can you sense a filling and emptying where you bring your attention? A subtle expansion and contraction? Continue to scan your body with this intention. Even if you don't sense the subtle breathing, you may be aware of a sense of aliveness, awakening, tingling, warmth, etc., as you bring your attention to each part, checking the shoulders, upper arms, elbows, forearms, wrists, hands, even each finger and toe. Can you sense the breath in your back, with the shifting of contact with the floor, mat, bed, back of the chair, or even your clothing? How much of the whole of your body can you sense at once?* Again, there is no right or wrong here. This is not a competition. This is about developing awareness. Begin by being aware of what you are aware of and what you are not aware of!

When you have explored this awareness of body sensations for a while, you may want to add a bit of movement. As you are lying or sitting, being aware of sensations in different parts of your body, what happens if you make some very tiny movements with your fingers? Start with one finger. The smaller the movement, the more likely you are to sense something in response to it. You may want to try making movements so small that someone observing you might not even see the motion, but you can feel it. *Can you sense even the intention of movement in your body? You may find you sense it not only in the finger moving but also in other parts of your body. Let yourself be curious. What can you sense? Where do you sense it? How much of the whole of your body can you be with in this exploration?* You can try this with various fingers, then progress to moving toes. Make the movements small, slow, and subtle. What happens? If you make larger, faster movements, you will have very different sensations. Try it if you like. You may find your breath becoming faster and your focus shifting. Subtler movements will facilitate settling your nervous system and enhance focus and awareness.

Once you have had some time to play with exploring your awareness of body sensations, it is time to increase the level of challenge and bring your sensory awareness into relationship with others.

Presence and Relationship

Have you noticed that your ability to be with your breath and sensations shifts when you come into relationship with another person? *Take a moment now to sense your breath again, as it moves in and out of your body, and to be aware of whatever sensations you are aware of. Once you have a sense of the flow of the breath, imagine a friend or family member walking in through the door. What happens with your breath? What happens with your awareness of it? Can you still feel the breath?*

Often there is a change in our breath when we encounter others. This may be a remnant of our animal nature, a need to sense the person with us to ascertain if we are safe or not. As our sympathetic fight-or-flight nervous system is activated to enable us to be alert enough to check out the other person, our breath usually accelerates. With our attention on the other person, however, we often lose track of our breath as we enter the relational field. What happens if we settle back into a sense of breath?

What is in the way of our being present in relationship in this moment? In this relationship? As practitioners, it is important for us to be as present as possible. It can be useful in developing presence to consider how our previous relationships may influence our ability to interact in the current one with our client. In being a relational therapist, we learn about the phenomena of transference and counter-transference.

Transference, a psychoanalytic term first described by Freud, refers to the unconscious perceiving and relating to a person in present time, like a therapist, boss, or romantic partner, as someone from the past, usually a parent or other authority figure from childhood. This is an unconscious effort to heal the old relationship. In therapy, transference occurs as the client tends to re-enact a relationship from the past with the therapist. An important aspect of psychoanalysis involves the therapist recognizing the transference and assisting the client in becoming aware of it. While this requires a degree of neutrality on the therapist's part, therapists also have unfinished business from their own childhoods. Counter-transference refers to a therapist reacting to a client as if to someone from the therapist's past. While craniosacral therapists are not psychoanalysts, a relatively neutral presence is also useful in Craniosacral Biodynamics. We aim to be as present as possible with our clients in part to provide this neutrality.

Are we present in this relationship or are we interacting or reacting as if we were in another relationship with someone else at a different time? We may have become very young, relating to an authority figure, parent, grandparent, sick sibling, etc. Or we may have become one of our parents or other older role models for caregiving from when we were younger. It may be useful to draw on what we learned from these role models, but doing so unconsciously can interfere with being present in this relationship and may lead to inappropriate behavior or interventions.

I am reminded of Frederick Leboyer's description in his book, *Birth without Violence*, of the sense of urgency in cutting the umbilical cord at birth as being a replay of the urgency at the birth attendant's own birth.[42] The usually unnecessary and premature cutting of this essential lifeline just as the baby is adjusting to breathing can perpetuate the wounding that the birth attendant was drawn to their profession to heal. The same can be true for craniosacral therapists, feeling an urgent need to fix our client's pain, to have them feel like something significant happened in the session, to act out of a need to be seen, approved, accepted, welcomed, appreciated, etc. The client in these counter-transference situations often leaves feeling unseen and unmet. The urgency of the practitioner's needs directing the treatment backfires and neither client nor therapist feels satisfied. This of course is complicated further by the client's transference onto the practitioner, expecting or perceiving them to be like someone from the client's past.

Our tendency to project and act from our own history often relates to unresolved issues or trauma from our past. As our early traumas tend to occur within relationship, they tend to re-emerge in a similarly intimate relational field, such as that between therapist and client. We will discuss later how they arise in clients and how we approach this in Craniosacral Biodynamics. Here, our focus is on our presence as practitioners and how our own history can obstruct our ability to simply be with our clients. We may be acting instead from an unconscious drive to know and heal our own past.

How can we become more present with our clients? The first step, which we have been practicing in this chapter, is to be more present with ourselves. In a way, presence is the essence of relationship. In the next chapter, we continue this journey of settling with ourselves and each other, as we explore the healing potential of deepening together into a state of being, and the effects of presence in the settling of the relational field in Craniosacral Biodynamics. In later chapters, we will look at how presence supports the unfolding of the inherent treatment plan through resonance. Presence facilitates a sense of safety and settling, which enables both practitioner and client to deepen under the surface waves related to life's conditions and traumas, returning to the wholeness and health supporting forces of the Breath of Life.

3

The Space Between

Nurturing the Relational Field

This social engagement system enables people to touch each other. We don't just walk up and touch someone; there's a whole interaction between the face, vocalizations, other bodily cues, to see if we feel safe with each other. Then we can touch.

—STEPHEN PORGES[43]

When client and practitioner first come together, a meeting between two beings begins. We each arrive with our own past interpersonal histories informing our perceptions, behaviors, and bodies. Initially, there is a natural biological inquiry as to who this other being may be. Like all animals, we are geared to evaluate strangers as to how safe or threatening they may be. As my mentor, Emilie Conrad, would say, we "sniff each other out" until we know enough about the other to know we are safe and can begin to settle. In this chapter, we explore this important settling of our "relational field" in biodynamic sessions.

Franklyn Sills recognized that the unfolding of the "inherent treatment plan" described by Becker actually begins with the relationship between client and practitioner.[44] We refer to this potentially healing space created between client and practitioner as the *relational field*. If the client does not feel safe in relationship to the practitioner within the field between them, the client's system will be challenged to settle under its defensive activation and the deeper biodynamic forces will be less easily perceived. Old patterned activities will tend to continue, designed as they are for survival and protection. In this habitual state, the client's system is oriented to conditions adapted to in the past, rather than to what is available in the present time. The inherent treatment plan unfolds when the system is able to settle and shift to a sense of wholeness, oriented to Primary Respiration. We will discuss this "holistic shift" more in the next chapter. For now it's important to note that it occurs only when the client experiences adequate trust and safety. The client's system can then begin to settle under its protective patterning, enabling it to orient to the healing potential offered by the current moment and relationship.

Our relationship with the client begins with our first contact. What we put out in our publicity—the client's relationship with and respect for the person who referred them to us, our first contact by telephone, email, etc.—are all important in creating the relational field in which the work can happen. Through our words, tone of voice, facial expressions, and behavior, we signal to the client how safe and welcoming, or threatening and frightening, we can be.

Whether we like to think of this or not, human beings are animals. We check (often unconsciously) if the other person is safe to be with. To what extent can we let down our guard and begin to relax? In many forms of bodywork, this is less essential, or at least less emphasized. Because Craniosacral Biodynamics works with deep, universal forces operating prior to and beyond our conditioning, we cannot proceed without attending to the therapeutic relationship. This makes sense when we consider where our conditioning comes from.

Our relational history begins within a family context. Our original patterning for how we interact with others is established as early as birth and even within the womb. The way we experience and are met, supported and reflected, or not, within our early primary relationships, affects our behavior and our experience of relationships throughout life. Bodywork involves physical proximity and contact, which may easily stimulate early memories from our first relationships, when we were similarly in close contact with another. While those memories are usually preverbal and often unconscious, our bodies tend to react as if they were recurring in present time. Horizontal on a treatment table with a practitioner hovering over us, doing things to us, can return us to the last time we were contacted in this way, often as a little one with mother or other caregivers.

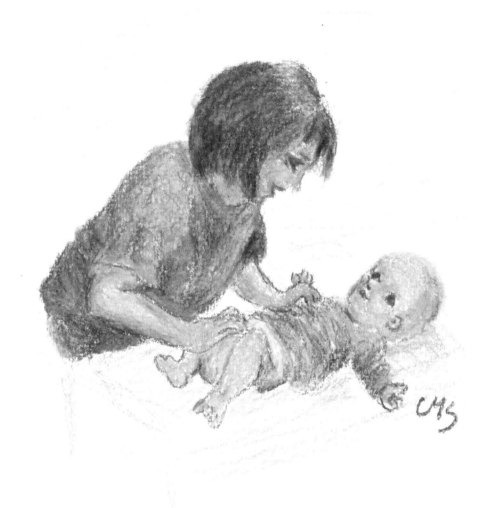

FIGURE 17: Infant on Table

In many forms of bodywork, talking is discouraged in favor of relaxation. As little ones, however, we may have had people doing things to us without explaining or checking in with us. For babies this can not only be disempowering, but also confusing, disorienting, and even terrifying. Moreover, infants and young children process information more slowly than adults as their nervous systems are still developing. A fast approach or transition can be overwhelming and shocking for them. Clients on the treatment table may re-enter a state like a little one, becoming nonverbal, helpless to respond, compliant in order to not be hurt or rejected, or frozen or dissociated to avoid feeling the discomfort. We will discuss this kind of reaction and how to work with it in Craniosacral Biodynamics more in chapter 7. For now, I want to emphasize that in Craniosacral Biodynamics it is essential to check in with the client in a relational way to help them to be present with us, in support of the inherent treatment plan being able to unfold. As indicated in chapter 2, we are more able to support our clients in being present with them and in meeting their needs in such a way that they can feel safe if we ourselves are present. If we are not aware of our own historical tendencies, we tend to act them out unconsciously in ways that are of service neither to ourselves as practitioners nor to our clients.

Source, Being, and Self

Our relational abilities are affected developmentally as our personalities develop. Sills refers to three states he terms source, being, and self. He writes, "These terms are derived from Buddhist concepts of *bodhicitta,* the already enlightened ground state; *citta,* the manifestation of that state as the core of our human existence; and *atta,* the self that is generated in response to life conditions. These are not mutually exclusive territories, but are holographically enfolded and spontaneously co-arise."[45]

Source is an inherently spiritual state, universal, open, nonjudgmental, and exists prior to and beyond our life conditioning. *Being* is the natural state of the little one. As noted in chapter 2, D. W. Winnicott emphasized the importance of an adequate empathic holding environment enabling the little one to have a "continuity of being" in an undefended state, protected by the caregiver from impingements.[46] In this state of being at any stage of life, we are open to and connected to source, an ultimate resource ("re-source"). As life's conditions set in, we learn how to act in more specific, socially acceptable ways. We develop a *self* state, formed by necessary defensive strategies and personality structures. When we relate to others from this *self,* or little ego self state, our perception of others is limited by our life experience, with its resultant beliefs, expectations, judgments, and needs. Clients often arrive in this state, consciously or unconsciously expecting the practitioner to perform in certain ways, or fearing they might re-enact behaviors experienced in past relationships. When we meet each other *self-to-self,* our relationships are determined by our histories. This is responsible for many issues intimate partners face, expressed as arguments, disillusionment, and often separation or divorce.

As Buddhist teacher, author, and psychologist Tara Brach points out, emotions are natural.[47] All animals apparently have them. What is different and problematic for humans is that we repetitively cycle and identify with our emotions through our special abilities to think about and analyze things. This identification is an aspect of self. While understanding can certainly be interesting and helpful, it can take us out of simply being. The arrows in figure 18 indicate different levels of relationship: self-to-self, self-to-being, and being-to-being.

If we are able to settle under and beyond our conditioned *self state,* we access a more harmonious, compassionate, empathetic *being state.* Here, sensing our support from source, we are less propelled by our own individual/self needs. We have a wider, more inclusive view, facilitating seeing the other person's perspective. Obviously, this is helpful for practitioners.

In Craniosacral Biodynamics, we utilize various practices to settle ourselves under our conditioning, so that we can meet clients from a state of being. This is akin to a reparenting process, where the client can be acknowledged, accepted, and received unconditionally, as every child needs. Here the work can begin to deepen within a settled relational field. Often, as the therapeutic relationship develops, clients who

Self-to-Self, Being-to-Self, and Being-to-Being Relationships

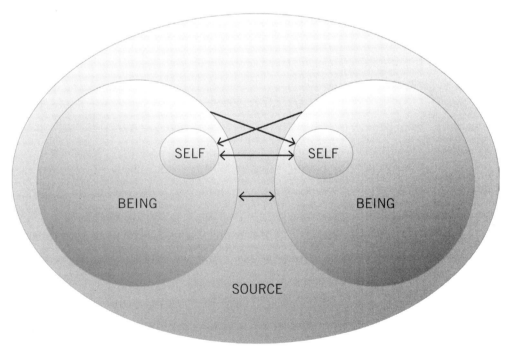

FIGURE 18: Source, Being, and Self in Relationship
Thanks to Franklyn Sills for inspiring the image. To read more on these concepts,
please refer to his book *Being and Becoming.*

begin in a self state are able to settle with us and our relationship shifts from being-to-self into being-to-being. Winnicott describes how "an environment we can rely upon allows us to establish a place we can retire to, to simply be."[48] Within such a context, our clients' natural potential can unfold, like little ones held with what Winnicott referred to frequently as "good-enough" mothering.[49] This chapter offers guidance and insight into how such a nurturing, holding environment is created through our relational settling process.

Being and Presence

The relational field begins before the first session, and actually before we even meet the client. If I as practitioner choose to meet my clients from a state of being, I need to nurture that state within myself, apart from actual session time with clients, so I can be in a being state when they arrive in my office.

As discussed in chapter 2, the professional Craniosacral Biodynamics practitioner training teaches student practitioners many different ways to settle into being within themselves. These include simple mindfulness practices, like observing the breath as it moves in and out of the body. *Can you sense yours now?* Generally, the more relaxed we are, the deeper the breath can move in the body and the more we can settle into being. Chest breathing tends to relate to a more activated, anxious, or speedy state, with a more active sympathetic nervous system. Belly breathing connects to a more settled nervous system state. The parasympathetic nervous system is functioning, supporting the breath in feeding the organs of digestion and reproduction, enabling rest and rejuvenation.

As mentioned in the last chapter, considering the purpose of the breath to carry oxygen to every cell in the body and carbon dioxide and other wastes away, we can acknowledge the possibility of every cell in the body breathing, and of sensing that. This kind of awareness requires slowing down, which takes us into more subtle realms of perception. We usually need to settle under a survival focus in order to perceive at this level. We explored this in chapter 2 but it is useful to revisit it here. *Take some time to observe your breath. Do you feel any slower after being with your breath? Did you notice your breath change at all as you were with it? How is it now? Can you read this page and be aware of your breath at the same time?*

Awareness is an essential aspect of presence. If you are with someone and thinking about your shopping list or what you are going to say next or where you are going after this meeting, you are not really present with them. Are you even present with yourself? Research indicates that healing, regardless of the therapy techniques involved, depends on the relationship between therapist and client. Presence enhances relationship.[50] *Have you ever been with someone and felt like they weren't really there with you? How was that for you? What do you sense in your body now as you remember this experience or type of experience?* You may find yourself withdrawing, your body contracting away from the person. What is the point of making an effort to connect with someone who isn't really there? You may even dissociate if you have a parasympathetic freeze tendency activated when you don't feel safe or welcomed. Alternatively, you may find yourself working extra hard to get this person to really respond to you. You need to feel they are there with you! The unsettledness of this experience may be accompanied by physiological changes as your animal body registers potential threat. Your sympathetics are activated, as is your attachment patterning from your childhood. Heart rate increases. Breathing becomes more rapid and shallow as you almost desperately search for ways to engage.

As I write this, I am reminded of my own childhood. My mother didn't feel very present to me. I now know from years of studying psychotherapy and trauma that she was highly dissociated due to her own history. She also was very drugged when I was born and was completely unconscious through most of the labor. This interfered with us being able to bond. As mentioned in chapter 2, I finally felt we bonded fifty years later! For a newborn, it can be terrifying to feel that lack of presence in the mother. The little one's survival depends on the caregiver being present and aware. For me, until I resolved this issue through my own therapy, that terror resurfaced when I was with people who were similarly dissociated. If people didn't feel present to me, I either avoided them or tried to support them in being able to be present. Interestingly, my life work is about teaching presence!

How is it for you to be here just now? How is it for you to read these words? Do they resonate at all for you? Are you aware of your self as you read? Do you sense your breath? Can you sense your body? Sensing bodily sensations is a major aspect of mindfulness practice, which we find essential in biodynamic practice. This somatic awareness not only supports the practitioner in being present, but, as you will see later, also facilitates awareness and healing in the client.

As we develop awareness of sensation, a sense of our feet on the floor, of our breath, of the weight of our body resting into the support of gravity, we begin to be able to settle into this moment more fully. It is as if this information reassures us that we are here, that we can be here because we are safe. If I feel the support of the earth under me, I can begin to settle into it and to arrive more fully. I can start to feel truly safe. With a sense of safety, we begin to settle. Our nervous system shifts from defensive fight, flight, or freeze states, and we find ourselves feeling more present, relaxed, and interactive. Neuroscientist Stephen Porges, who proposed a new way of viewing the autonomic nervous system with his Polyvagal Theory mentioned in chapter 2, points out that our perception changes as we shift out of defensive states into what he terms the social engagement system.[51] Here, we are neurologically able to perceive safety in present time, rather than reacting as if past danger were following us. In Craniosacral Biodynamics, we aim to be in this state as practitioners and to support our clients in being able to settle in this way with us.

Resting in Resource

When clients arrive, they are often in a relatively activated state. In the modern Western world, the very process of arriving can be speedy and overstimulating. Life itself can be overwhelming! As I write this chapter, I sit in a public library in New York City. Although libraries are relatively quiet, this one, like everything in this city, is full of people. There are literally people everywhere! There is not much talking, except at the information desk, but I am surrounded by the tapping of computer keys, the ringing of mobile phones, the scraping of chairs being moved, as well as intermittent coughing, clearing of throats, and occasionally the slamming of doors and clicking of loud heels. This is a quiet place in the city! On the street outside, my nervous system is bombarded by the sounds of traffic, sirens, honking, talking, and music. There are flashing neon signs, and in fact signs everywhere you look, faces, movement, colorful clothing, too much to possibly take in at any given moment. I compare this to the quiet little Elizabethan market town where I live in England. There I can say hello to rabbits, sheep, and cows on my daily walk. Even there, however, people rush to appointments, get stuck in traffic, are distracted by shopping, etc. In our modern world, we are rarely free of stimulation, and most of it is fast and frequent. No matter how well I understand this, my animal nervous system still reacts, seeking to evaluate how safe or threatened I may be in any given moment. How can I rest in the midst of all of this?

Rest is possible when my system has the ability to be with what it encounters. Overwhelm involves too much input for what the system can handle. For example, trying to be aware of everything is generally too much to process. Those of us with a history of trauma may find ourselves being hypervigilant, distracted by every little sound, every movement we detect out the corner of the eye, and every change in our environment. There may have been a time when our survival depended on such astute awareness. We may have needed to know when to expect the next attack in order to protect ourselves. Settling becomes difficult with this kind of history until we learn to hone our attention to what is actually present and relevant now.

What tells me I am safe now? I can feel my breath. This tells me I am alive. Where there is life, there is hope. I can feel my feet. This tells me I have the ground under me. There is some support. Mindful awareness brings me or the client into present time, actually shifting our neurobiology. Visual awareness may also be helpful. Looking around the room, I see the shapes and colors of this present-day room. I practice being aware of what is now. I may hear sounds from outside, but I know I have not been attacked in many years. As I allow myself to listen, I hear these are the sounds of traffic, or of squirrels, or whatever it actually is. I can begin to feel safe and rest again. Rest can arrive through awareness of what is present here and now.

For some, however, this shift of focus is too big a step. Sounds in the distance always mean danger. There is no sense of safety. Nonetheless, we all have resources, or things that support us in the midst of our experience and help us to find a sense of safety and well-being. When we begin work with clients in Craniosacral Biodynamics, we generally check in as to how the person is and then guide them in orienting to resource. I might simply ask, what supports you in the midst of all this?

Shifting our perception as we shift our neurobiology has been studied since 1991 by the research organization HeartMath, mentioned in chapter 2. A booklet published by HeartMath states, "Current evidence suggests that this self-regulatory capacity relies on an inner resource akin to energy, which is used to interrupt the stream of information and behavior and alter it."[52] For a person affected by trauma or overwhelm, energy is taken up habitually to protect against the feelings or recurrence of the pain of the experience. The nervous system repeatedly returns to the upset introduced by that experience, requiring extra effort to attend to input from present time, such as the information that we are currently safe. Practice can establish a new baseline, rendering the new patterns of self-regulation automatic and not requiring as much energy expenditure, as our sense of inner resource grows.

The term *resource* can refer to all the things that support us in our lives, enabling us to cope and to experience well-being. Somatic Experiencing practitioners Diane Poole Heller and Larry Heller note that resource can be "anything that makes you feel safe and comfortable, helps discharge your tension or arousal, and triggers a relaxation response."[53] They help to build and balance the inner energy levels. Resources may include favorite possessions, clothing, jewelry, toys, pets, friends, family, hobbies, places, or activities, or memories or thoughts of any of these. These are examples of external resources, things outside ourselves that support us. If someone is unable to call to mind an external resource, one option is to imagine or visualize one, like an imaginary place where we can feel safe and nurtured, or the memory of a safe person, like a grandmother or other being from the past, or a spiritual being, that gives a sense of support. We also have internal resources, including qualities like strength, intelligence, ability to concentrate, warmth, friendliness, special talents, etc. Our physical sensations can also serve as resources.

In working with clients, we may begin by explaining this concept of resource and asking about what the person finds resourcing. We intend to begin our work on the treatment table from as settled a state as possible. Thinking and talking about resources tends to have a calming effect. For some people, asking about resource doesn't help. They have a hard time thinking of anything that resources them and feel worse because of this. They may, however, be supported by a comment about a beautiful piece of jewelry, or guidance in attending to their breath or their feet. For some, the act of talking itself is settling; for others it is unsettling. The intention is not so much talking about resource as it is to be oriented to resource, instead of just to whatever trauma or difficulty the person arrives with. We may need to be creative in helping clients access their resources and develop awareness of this process and its benefits. With children I may not talk about the concept of resource, but might remind them of one of their favorite things, which I learn about when interviewing their parents or through the child's behavior. If a child brings a cuddly toy with them, it's a good guess that this is a resource. Demonstrating interest in the toy helps draw attention to it and its resourcing effects. Usually, hopefully, the parent is also a resource for the child. I support them in going to the parent for comfort as needed

Please take a moment now to consider your own resources. I suggest taking a piece of paper and making two lists, "My External Resources" and "My Internal Resources." Take a few minutes to add some items to your lists. As you consider these resources, take note of how your body feels. How is your breath now? Do you feel more activated or more settled? What sensations tell you this?

It is common when accessing a resource for people to report feeling more settled. Words like *softer, melted, relaxed, calmer, warmer, smoother,* and *grounded* are common. There may be more awareness lower in the body, like the feet on the floor or the body making contact with the chair or treatment table. Often the breath becomes deeper, slower, and easier. The person begins to speak more slowly, and awareness comes into this moment and this relationship. What we call the relational field begins to feel more settled. This is a starting point for Craniosacral Biodynamics.

Relational Field and Trust

The term *relational field* as used in Craniosacral Biodynamics was borrowed from Core Process Psychotherapy as developed by Maura Sills, assisted by Franklyn Sills, starting in the 1980s.[54] The concept of the relational field is influenced by the work of psychoanalyst Donald Winnicott, who wrote of the importance of a "good-enough holding environment" for little ones.[55] Here, the mother or other caregiver is sufficiently attuned and responsive to the child, protecting them from impingements, enabling them to remain in a state of being. Winnicott also addressed the space between mother and child, as did Martin Buber, who wrote in his treatise *I and Thou,* "In the beginning is relation—as category of being, readiness, grasping form, mould for the soul: it is the *a priori* of relation, *the inborn Thou.*"[56]

Life falters without relationship. For example, failure to thrive can occur when babies are neglected and deprived of the relational holding they depend on.[57] We now know that little ones' brain and nervous system development depend on safe, nurturing social interaction with their caregivers. From an epigenetic perspective, we also understand that genes are turned on and off in relationship to the environment, including the people around them.[58] Babies in the womb are preparing on a genetic level for the world they will come more fully into at birth, and they learn about this through their mother's emotional states and perceptions before birth. If Mom perceives her world as safe and nurturing, baby prepares to enter into a safe, nurturing world. If Mom's perception is that she is not safe and nurtured, her baby develops accordingly, tending to be physiologically more attuned to stress, with more development of the soma that can support fight-or-flight responses and less development of the areas of the brain involved with reasoning and social interaction.[59] Our bodies, brains, and even cells develop, grow, and communicate within relationship. This begins at conception within the context of the parental relational field and continues throughout life.

As with practitioner and client, the relationship between mother and baby is essential to life. For babies, this is about survival. For our clients it is usually more about thriving, coming more fully into the potential life offers, embodying fuller life energy.

Where clients have experienced a threatening environment, they may function and perceive life and relationships as if they were about survival. They need to learn that a different kind of relationship is possible. In Craniosacral Biodynamics, we aim to provide a safe, nurturing relational field, a context different from the unsafe one of the past, where trust can emerge within a sense of safe holding.

Gabor Maté, a physician who sees many medical issues as being made possible by early environment, writes in this vein on attention deficit disorder, "The answer to underdevelopment is development, and for development the appropriate conditions must exist...We may not be able to prescribe development directly, but we can promote an environment that makes development possible."[60]

A safe relational field is an environment with appropriate conditions for the development of what has not been nurtured to develop in the past and to heal what has needed to emerge in response to the conditions that have existed in life. This may be on a psychological as well as a physical level.

Describing the effects of one's relational field, Winnicott writes, "The potential space between baby and mother, between child and family, between individual and society and the world, depends on experience which leads to trust. It can be looked upon as sacred to the individual, in that it is here that the individual experiences creative living."[61]

Where the trust has not been established in the early mother–child or equivalent relationship, or trust has later been betrayed, there is usually a need to rebuild it within the therapeutic relationship. It is essential for practitioners to provide a *good-enough* holding environment, such as the little one needed initially with mother.[62] This becomes a foundation for the development of trust, openness and relaxation. Note that it is not necessary, and perhaps not even beneficial (or possible) to be perfect in every way. We need only to be "good enough." This means that the child, or client, feels heard, seen, and met in a relatively consistent way. Where we miss, repair is essential. I remember working with an eight-week-old baby once who seemed to be doing very well. At one point in our craniosacral session, I suddenly realized he was showing me his birth, as little ones often do. He had some feelings about this event, even though everyone thought it had been a beautiful, easy birth. After he had expressed his feelings by crying as he rotated and pushed through a remembered birth canal, I apologized to him. I said something to the effect that I was sorry that I hadn't realized these feelings were here and that I hadn't understood this right away. He looked at me

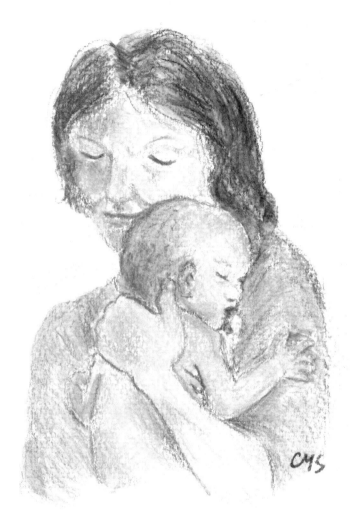

FIGURE 19: Mother and Child

for a moment and then began to laugh! Both his parents insisted that he thought my apology was hilarious. He was clearly very happy and ready to accept it!

There are always going to be times when we don't quite get what is being asked of us or expressed to us. We may make an assumption about the client's needs based on the last few sessions. Or we may just be human. It is important to put aside our pride and acknowledge to the client, as with children, that we have made a mistake or didn't quite get it right.

It is within such a relational field that defensive neural patterning can begin to settle as the social engagement system comes forward, facilitating relational interaction in present time. In support of this, biodynamic practitioners intend to meet their clients from a heart-centered receptive state, settling themselves in stillness and being.

Franklyn Sills writes,

> In craniosacral biodynamics, we learn to generate a holding field rooted in presence and being. From this ground, we hold the client in a wide and soft perceptual field oriented to inherent Health via an awareness of primary respiration within both our own system and the client's. This then deepens into an appreciation of the Stillness from which being emerges and the universal Source that supports all life. As this clarifies, genuine interconnection is sensed that is not an expression of either the practitioner or client's conditioned experience. Empathy is a function of this connection. It is a natural outflow of compassion in the presence of suffering, being-to-being. It is this that allows the practitioner to appropriately respond to the actual state of the client and to unconditionally accept their presence. The first step in any healing process is the settling of the relational field into a state of basic trust. This is directly sensed as a mind-body settling within and between both practitioner and client.[63]

Space, Contact, and Respect

Winnicott described elements of the good-enough holding environment as holding, handling, and object presentation.[64] All of these are relevant in biodynamic practice. We keep them in mind when making physical and energetic contact with the client. Our intention is always to support settling and deepening within our relational field.

When we make physical contact with clients, we let them know we are about to do so, or check to make sure they are ready for it. Our intention is to not startle them when we make or shift contact. Many clients have had negative experiences with touch previously. They may have had parents or other caregivers who were not sensitive in their approach and handling when they were little. They may have been physically or sexually abused by parents, teachers, or others. Unfortunately, they may have received bodywork previously that felt invasive or abusive to them, or the bodyworker may have had inappropriate boundaries. Even if they were too young or traumatized to consciously remember early incidents, the body remembers and may react to new contact as if the past were happening again.

This dynamic may be exacerbated by the position of the client, lying horizontal on the treatment table. This position is reminiscent of how babies spend much of their time, as well as how sexual abuse may occur. It may also stimulate somatic memories of being ill and dependent in the hospital, possibly medicated and unable to actively protect oneself. Lying down on the treatment table with a practitioner poised over the client may trigger memories of frightening or dangerous past experiences. In this situation, clients often shift automatically into defensive neural pathways. They may become activated, ready to jump off the table and run out the room if their sympathetic, flight-or-fight nervous system is stimulated. Or, they may suddenly go into a parasympathetic freeze state. We will look at this more in chapter 7. At this point, I want to note that where there is unresolved trauma in a person's system, the trauma may resurface and interfere with settling within the relational field. Just being with another person may be enough to trigger this activation. In Craniosacral Biodynamics, there is the potential to be present in a relatively intimate way, with several elements of the session possibly resembling challenging past events. Where there has been trauma, we cannot assume we are beginning a session with trust already available in the relational field. We often need to seed and grow the trust between us.

Simple acts like letting the client know we are about to make contact can help to establish trust and a sense of safety. Once we have made contact, we want to check with the client that the contact is comfortable. I explain to new clients that in this work, client comfort is extremely important, because the work depends on settling and it's harder to relax if you are uncomfortable. To this end, I explain that I will be letting them know when I shift contact and will check as to how comfortable the contact is each time. I ask them to please tell me if anything at all is uncomfortable because we can probably adjust something to make it more comfortable. This may take some educating. So many of us have been trained to not complain, to not ask for what we need, or to not even notice if we need something. Speaking or expressing our discomfort may have been discouraged, dangerous, or even life-threatening in past situations. Learning to communicate our needs is an aspect of a safe, respectful relational field.

Relating within Resonant Fields

Establishing a comfortable physical contact involves energetic as well as physical negotiation. In Craniosacral Biodynamics, we sense into this energetic distance between practitioner and client, and may verbally ask the client to explore with us a different energetic contact as we intend more or less space. We will look at how to do this soon, but first it is helpful to understand that the space between us includes an energetic space, where our energetic fields overlap.

Science is now demonstrating what healers have sensed for eons: We are energetic beings. Our bodies communicate with each other via vibration. As Lynne McTaggart states in her book *The Field*, "The vibration of one body is reinforced by the vibration of another body at or near its frequency."[65] We sense each other's vibratory presence naturally. Have you ever walked into a party and felt instantly attracted to someone? Or repulsed? We tend to want to be close to those whose vibrations are more like ours (resonant) and to avoid those whose energy is different (dissonant). Or we may be attracted to someone who resonates with our history, represented by an aspect within us. For example, how many of us have seemingly married our father or mother? We may think we are different from our parents, but usually we have developed our sense of who we are in relation to them. Even if we have made ourselves the complete opposite of our parents, they remain the reference point for that opposition. When we are attracted to someone like one of our parents, there is generally a resonance between that person and the aspect of us that is energetically like our parents. We are unconsciously seeking what is familiar, which can be reassuring and comfortable. If this relates to our past relationships, an opportunity for healing is also available. When we bring conscious awareness to what is familiar, our patterns can begin to shift. We may then begin to resonate with different people. In any case, we tend to be drawn to each other energetically through resonance. In this vein, clients often choose a practitioner based on their sense of energetic resonance. They come back to us because they feel comfortable. We want to support that sense of resonance, as it can facilitate relational field settling and healing.

Understanding our energetic nature can enhance our ability to contribute to a beneficially resonant relational field. Why are we so energetically connected? We are apparently all connected via an energetic "Zero Point Field."[66] Via this field, we can affect one another with our presence and our consciousness. For example, groups of meditators intending specific changes toward health in a specific target person appear to have exactly the intended effect.[67] McTaggart, author of *The Field, The Bond, The Intention Experiment, and The Power of Eight,* has been overseeing such experiments based on Web participation by thousands of people, with promising results. Such studies suggest an important relational resonance inherent in hands-on healing modalities. Similarly, James Oschman, in his book *Energy Medicine: The Scientific Basis*, discusses energy healing modalities as involving entrainment or resonance between practitioner and client.[68] HeartMath researchers have concluded that we communicate with and sense one another via our hearts' magnetic fields, and that this ability is enhanced in a state of coherence.[69]

The significance of vibrational resonance is perhaps less obscure when we consider that we are composed primarily of water. Our bodies have been said to be about 70 percent water as adults.[70] We begin as highly fluid beings, with a tendency to become drier as we age, ranging from 96 percent water as a fertilized egg, to 80 percent in the infant, to 70 percent in adults, and 60 percent in the average elderly person.[71] Water is a highly resonant element. The work of Japanese researcher Masaru Emoto beautifully demonstrates how water can pick up the vibratory messages of words. Emoto photographed crystalized water that had been exposed to words like *love, thanks,* and *I hate you,* as well as different kinds of music. The crystals photographed looked very different depending on the kind of words or music presented.[72] While Emoto's research has been questioned and difficult to replicate, another researcher, William Tiller, has demonstrated how water responds to human intention, measured by the effects of meditators' intentions to raise or lower the pH of water, even at a distance.[73]

If water responds to such intentions, and we are made up mostly of water, we can understand that our clients' bodies will also respond to our intentions as practitioners. Indeed, Tiller has also studied how meditators' focused intention can reduce anxiety and depression in research subjects.[74] It seems inherent in our human being-ness to be energetically sensitive to the presence and intentions of others. As fluid, energetic beings, we all participate in a continuum. Emilie Conrad, founder of Continuum Movement, pointed out that "all fluids, whether in the cell, the body, or the planet, function as a resonant intelligent whole and can never be separated"[75] Your fluid body and mine are intimately connected on an energetic, vibrational level. Cells, made up mostly of fluid, oscillate and resonate. Our health depends on intercellular communication within and between individuals. We are engaged in an ongoing dance with all other fluid, oscillatory beings, bodies, and the cosmos as a whole.

In Craniosacral Biodynamics, we are particularly aware of the extreme sensitivity of the fluid body we are making contact with. We do our best to negotiate our physical and energetic contact with careful respect, acknowledging the person who may feel as vulnerable as a little infant within an exquisitely aware and responsive body. Our intentions as practitioners must be as conscious as possible. It is not unusual for beginner student practitioners in their eagerness to learn to sense the subtle rhythms we work with or the relevant anatomy to narrow their focus in on the desired object. In response, the client often feels pressure, which is the pressure of the practitioner's intention. Clients may complain of pain, restlessness, or other activation as the innocent novice practitioner is energetically pressing in on the client's field with a need to sense or find a particular phenomenon. I remind students at this point to widen and soften their attention, a practice emphasized as an essential foundational skill in the practitioner training.

I also suggest again that being with a client can be like going into the forest in search of wild animals. If we go clambering in, making noise, moving leaves and branches to meet our intention, we are not likely to see any animals. Intelligently defensive, they will hide until the threatening intrusion quiets down. If we sit quietly, however, allowing ourselves to just take in the scene, we may soon find ourselves delighted by an audience of curious animals. Meeting a client's system is similar. It will retreat if we are too brash and noisy in pursuit of our intentions. When we settle ourselves, the client's system begins to resonate with ours. It is as if we remind the client's system of what it is capable of. It begins to settle too. We begin to sense the activation quieting. As we are perceived as safe, the rhythms or anatomy we hoped to encounter are then more likely to present. The intentions of the client's system can then begin to surface, as the inherent treatment plan is expressed.

Exploring Your Relational Field

This section offers several exercises similar to those used in our practitioner trainings to explore and inquire into your experience within a relational field. The first exercises can be done on your own, with your imagination. For the others, you will need a friend or colleague as a partner. You may want to record these instructions in your own voice to listen to with your eyes closed, or you can alternate reading the instructions and exploring your experience. (Recordings are available at www.birthingyourlife.org /the-breath-of-life-book.)

Being with Self, Being with Other

Begin by sitting quietly in a comfortable position. As you settle yourself, notice what sensations are guiding you in the process. As you are moving your body to get comfortable, what sensations tell you to move? What tells you that you are comfortable or not? Can you sense the shifting of the weight of your body and the places where your body makes contact with the floor, cushion, chair, or whatever you are sitting on? As you settle, can you sense your breath? Where and how do you sense it in your body? How fast or slow is it? What sensations speak to you of settling? Perhaps the breath becomes slower and softer. You may have a sense of the sensations of your body coming more into focus, becoming more available.

Once you have a sense of being settled, allow yourself to imagine someone entering the room. What happens to your breath? What happens to your sense of being settled? Imagine for a moment that this person is a stranger to you. What happens with your breath and sensations? Now imagine this person is a dear friend or family member you are delighted to see. How does this affect your breath and body sensations? Do they change in some way? Does your access to breath and sensations, your ability to sense them, change in some way? Can you feel your face? Do you have a sense of it lighting up in some way? Or the expression on it changing? How does your heart feel? When you feel you have explored this sufficiently for a few minutes, take a little time to open your eyes, to look around the room to orient yourself. Notice how your breath and body are as you do this.

Take some notes on this experience to refer back to.

The next part requires a partner. *Take some time to sit quietly with your partner, repeating the exercise above that you did with yourself, checking in with your breath, your body sensations, your heart. Does anything feel any different from how it was when you were on your own? If so, how is it different? Take some notes about how this experience is for you; then take some time to share with your partner about your experience. After this sharing, return to sitting quietly together, observing your breath and body again. Has anything changed after having talked with your partner? Feel free to share with your partner what you discover.*

Negotiating Energetic Space and Distance

This is another partner exploration. *Begin by standing facing your partner. One of you will be A and one will be B. A is going to stay in place while B moves forward and back very slowly, checking in with A as to how this distance feels. As you do this, both of you check into your breath and body sensations, as well as emotions, verbally communicating with each other about what you are experiencing. When you find the distance that feels right, let each other know that. You may want to experiment a bit further, going a little closer or farther than feels right, then back to what does feel right. Once you are satisfied with your explorations, sit down. Check into your breath and body in this new position. You may find that sitting changes how close or far apart you want to be. Adjust your distance as feels right to you both, repeating the exercise in sitting. When you both feel you have found the right distance between you, take some time to just settle there together. How is it to sit together in this way? How does this compare to how it was for you in the previous exercise? What is your sense of the relational field between you? Do you have a sense of your partner being present with you and you being present with your partner? How is that for you?*

These explorations can be useful for learning about your style and tendencies in relationship, as well as for developing presencing skills in relation to another person. As you did these exercises, did your ability to sense your own breath and body change at all? Often, people find that their sense of their breath and sensation is more difficult to find when with another person. It is as if all their attention is drawn out toward the other person. This can relate to the need to gather information about the other person in order to feel safe. It is of course important to know that we are safe. If, however, all of your attention goes to the other person, it is possible to miss the signs in your own body also offering important information. For example, if I am with someone I don't feel safe with, my heart rate may increase as my sympathetic nervous system becomes activated, preparing me to fight or flee. Focusing all my attention on the other person, I may not notice how my own system has accelerated. I may also be less aware of my own intuitive sense of the other person, which communicates with me through body sensation.

In Craniosacral Biodynamics, it is particularly important when making contact with clients to be aware of your own relational tendencies and to prevent them from influencing the session. The tendency to reach out toward the other person can be read by a client's system as an intrusive force, needing to be protected against or adapted to. The entire session may revolve around this defensive reaction, interfering with settling and emergence of the intentions of the inherent treatment plan. Similarly, you may find your tendency when with another person is to withdraw within yourself. This too is a protective defensive stance, designed to avoid being hurt or attacked by the other person. These defensive habits are based on past relational experiences. They reduce our ability to just be present with the other, or to simply be. Clients of a practitioner in withdrawal often feel unmet. Energetically, they may reach out searching for the practitioner. Unfortunately, I have heard of and witnessed people practicing Craniosacral Therapy in a dissociative state where they are not actually present in relationship with the client. The practitioner may enjoy lovely images or a sense of light or what they believe is long tide, but they are actually not present. Again, clients may feel unmet in this situation.

As practitioners, we learn to sense when a client needs or wants closer energetic contact and how to adjust our energetic distance in support of the client being energetically met. This requires a degree of neutrality on the part of the practitioner. Awareness of our tendencies is a first step in liberating ourselves from their hold. As we develop awareness, we become more able to make other choices and expand our repertoire of behavior. Learning to be present with our own historical reactions can lead to profound healing. Often, therapeutic support in this process is helpful. Wounding that has occurred within relationship tends to heal most readily within a relational field. This is one aspect of the healing available from biodynamic sessions, where we have an intention for safety, nurturance, and support for the client.

Physical Contact within the Relational Field

Biodynamic sessions involve physical as well as energetic contact. In support of safety and settling, we negotiate the contact, rather than just putting our hands somewhere or removing them without warning. The next exercises involve this kind of negotiation. (Recordings are available at www.birthingyourlife.org/the-breath-of-life-book.)

In the first exploration, you will make some contact with your own body and sense into it. *Begin by sitting quietly as before, checking in with your breath and body sensations, including listening for a minute or two to your heart. Once you have settled this way with yourself, lift your hands and rub the palms together for a minute or so. Then, move your hands about a foot (thirty centimeters) apart, palms facing each other. Slowly bring them toward each other. At some point, do you sense the energy between them? It may feel like warmth, or buzzing. It may feel like you hit a barrier that takes effort to move beyond. Let yourself be curious. We are energetic entities. We can sense the energy of our bodies. How do you sense this? How far apart are your hands when you sense it? Feel free to repeat the exercise, rubbing your hands together again, to enhance your sense of the energy. This can be particularly helpful if you don't have a very strong sense of it.*

When you feel satisfied with this exploration, begin to bring one hand slowly toward your thigh. Do you have any sense of the energy coming off your thigh? Does your thigh sense the approach of your hand in any way? For example, you may feel its warmth, or a slight pressure. When it feels right, allow your hand to make physical contact with your leg. Notice how you know when it feels right. What are the sensations like that tell you it is right? Or not? Is your hand in the right place? If not, move it slightly until the placement feels right. How do you sense that rightness or the lack of it? Next, experiment with the quality of the contact you are making. Press into your leg with your hand a bit more. How does that increased contact feel? Lighten your pressure and check how that feels. Find the contact that feels just right. How do you know it is right? What sensations are guiding you?

You can also adjust the energetic space within your contact. *Once you have the right physical contact, imagine moving your attention closer to your hand, without changing it physically. Just as you moved closer to and farther from your partner previously, you can move your attention closer and farther. Imagine moving your attention back away from your leg. How does that feel?* Often, when clients aren't comfortable with our contact, the physical contact is right, but they need more energetic space. Moving your attention back can be helpful. Widening your attention can also help. *With your hand still on your leg, experiment with how it feels when you think of widening your attention. This isn't about going so wide that you lose touch with your own body. Instead, let yourself be aware of the center of your body and widen your awareness without losing a sense of that center.*

In Craniosacral Biodynamics, we work with what we call the midline, a still space running lengthwise through the center of the body. One way to begin to have a sense of midline is to think about your spine, a physical midline. *Let your awareness be centered in the area of your spine, and begin to widen it out toward the edges of your body. How wide can your awareness go without losing a sense of your own midline or spine? You may find you can widen your attention beyond the edges of your physical body, out toward the edges of the room you are in, or even toward the horizon.* It takes practice to be able to do this without losing your sense of yourself and your own midline. In that the work is relational, it is important to stay present with yourself. Relationship happens between two people. If one of them isn't present, there isn't really a relationship!

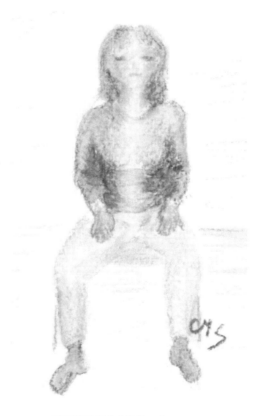

FIGURE 20A: Midline Awareness

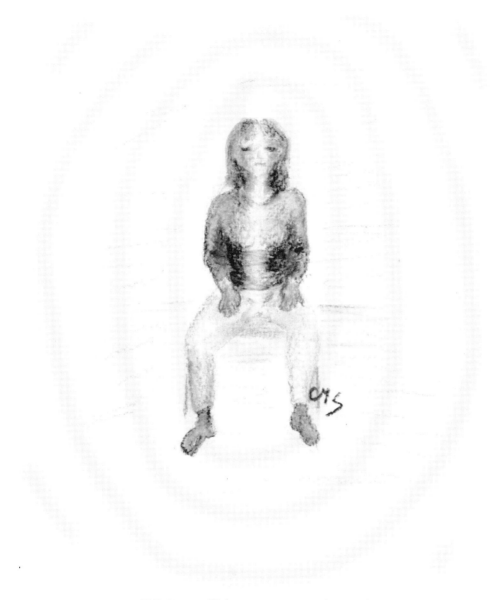

FIGURE 20B: Widening Awareness out from Midline

Take a little time to practice this widening of awareness while staying with your sense of your spine or midline. Then practice it while sensing how it affects your sense of your hand on your leg. Can you feel changes as you shift your attention? As you widen and narrow your attention, or bring it out from and in toward your leg, you are shifting the energetic space within the contact. Find the distance that feels right to you. Again, what sensations tell you this feels right? This is an exercise in shifting our mode of perception. We tend to learn in our modern Western world to narrow our attention, to focus in on whatever it is we are interested in. While this may be useful in gathering detailed information, it can feel intrusive if we focus on a client in this way. It can also interfere with our ability to sense the whole of the person, including the energetic field phenomena important in Craniosacral Biodynamics. As we practice widening our perception, we begin to find ourselves sensing more of the whole. Subtle energetic rhythms of life then tend to naturally become part of our vista.

As you are developing this ability to rest within a wider field of perception, you may find it easier making contact with your own body. The next step is to explore this negotiated contact with a partner. *Begin by sitting next to each other in a position where both of you are comfortably supported and you can easily rest your hand on your partner's thigh or arm. Ask your partner to show you where to put your hand. Take some time to sit quietly together and settle into a sense of breath and sensations as before. Then ask your partner if they are ready for you to make contact. If yes, let them know you are beginning to bring your hand to the spot chosen on their leg or arm. Begin moving your hand very slowly toward the place chosen for contact. Check in with each other verbally as to what you are both sensing as you bring your hand in. Be careful to keep your attention wide, rather than narrowing it in toward your partner.*

Can you sense each other's energy? How does it feel? Once you have made contact, play with the firmness or lightness of the contact, as you did with your own leg. Share with each other what you sense as you shift, and have your partner tell you when it feels right. Then, as you did with your leg, begin to experiment with your energetic distance, moving your attention in and out, widening out from your midline or narrowing back in toward it. Share how this feels for each of you as you make each shift. Again, ask your partner to let you know when it feels right. *How does it feel to you?* Once you have reached this sense of rightness, take a few minutes to just settle together, just being quiet. *How does this feel? What are you both aware of?* When you feel done, let your partner know you are going to remove your hand; then slowly disengage your contact, sensing whatever you both sense through this process. Take some time to share with your partner about your experience. Reverse roles and repeat.*

This is essentially how we make contact in Craniosacral Biodynamics, although there are many aspects of what we may perceive. *How is this way of making contact for you? What have you learned through this process about your own relational tendencies? How easy or difficult was it for you to sense changes as you shifted contact and energetic space?* Exercises like this can give you information as to what areas may be easy or challenging for you relationally, suggesting where you can benefit from more practice and possibly therapeutic support.

How we enter into relationship and contact sets the ground for the healing work of Craniosacral Biodynamics to emerge. I have been touched by how profoundly these initial steps in settling the relational field and making contact can affect both clients and practitioners. I have had clients respond with tears of awe and gratitude when I ask them how the contact is for them. They tell me, "No one has ever asked me that before. No one has ever cared!" I care. The clients perceive and understand this. It may take some adjusting to, and that in itself can be a healing process. In the next chapter, we begin to look at what emerges as the relational field settles. As we deepen under the effects of history and life conditions, something profound becomes apparent. Sutherland called it the Breath of Life, and its manifestation during our lives, Primary Respiration.

4
Primary Respiration

An Introduction to Rhythms, Tides, and the Three Bodies

There is no drop of water in the ocean, not even in the deepest parts of the abyss, that does not know and respond to the mysterious forces that create the tide.

—RACHEL CARLSON, *The Sea Around Us*

In the later part of his life, William Sutherland, father of Cranial Osteopathy, spoke of the Breath of Life, a sacred presence generating what he called "Primary Respiration." This is different from the breath of air, or secondary respiration, that moves through our lungs. Craniosacral Biodynamics has evolved from Sutherland's perceptions and attempts to describe the manifestations and work of this mysterious Breath of Life and the Primary Respiration it generates.

In Craniosacral Biodynamics, we perceive Primary Respiration arising from a ground of dynamic stillness, from which we sense emerging an extremely slow, subtle undercurrent we call the groundswell. Primary Respiration manifests as a very slow rhythmic phenomenon we call long tide, and a somewhat faster, more embodied tide, called fluid tide, or mid-tide. The long tide arises from the groundswell to support specific expressions of form and life. We perceive these tides as breathing within energetic fields or bodies, termed the tidal body or field of long tide, and the fluid body or field related to mid-tide. It is as if the denser physical body, a field of cells and tissues, is suspended within the fluid field, which in turn is suspended within the tidal field, all suspended within the ground of dynamic stillness. In this chapter, we begin to explore this three-body suspensory system and how Primary Respiration expresses within it.

Primary Respiration

Imagine a great breath blowing in from afar, swirling, spiraling in toward the center of your being, drawing your spirit in with it, gathering the fluid it encounters into alignment, as it takes on form in relation to a center line. Like the embryo differentiating into form, this wind and its fluid spirals direct our cells into a shape increasingly resembling the human body as we know it. This is your body, emerging out of space, energy, and fluid into a coherent cellular-tissue field we call physical. Resonant with fluid systems everywhere, echoing the birth of new stars, galaxies, and planets, this enfolding characterizes development in the womb and continues to regenerate us throughout life. This is a process I sense with my hands on a client in a Biodynamic Craniosacral Therapy session.

We perceive the Breath of Life arising out of a depth of stillness and supporting all of creation. It generates vast ordering forces that organize galaxies, solar systems, planets, and life. Sutherland oriented to a primary ordering principle, a "Primary Respiration," generated by the Breath of Life. Primary Respiration, in essence, is a stable ordering force, apparently moving from the horizon all around, toward and away from a person's center. It generates local ordering fields and manifests in an embodied fashion within the fluids of a person's system as a specific and essential form of bioenergy or life force. Sutherland called this embodied principle "potency." Potency manifests within the fluids of the embryo and is present as a fundamental organizing principle throughout life. This is similar to the understanding in Chinese philosophy of the *jing*, a coalescence of "cosmic chi" within a person's fluids, which has ordering, protective, and healing functions. We will discuss these functions of potency more in the next chapter on the inherent treatment plan.

A highly spiritual man, Sutherland took the term "the Breath of Life" from the Bible: "And the LORD God formed man *of* the dust of the ground, and breathed into his nostrils the breath of life; and man became a living soul."[76] Interestingly, immediately preceding this verse is one about water, also highly relevant to Craniosacral Therapy: "But there went up a mist from the earth, and watered the whole face of the ground."[77]

Once water was present on Earth, it became alive with plants and other living things. Like other living entities, humans can only emerge within a fluid environment.

Not only did the earliest creatures develop within the ocean, but humans continue in this vein, developing as embryos within fluid inside our mothers. Our conception can only occur within fluid, and we are nourished by the fluids around and within us as little ones in the womb and throughout our lives. We are made up primarily of water and, without it, we die, usually within a few days. Founder of Osteopathy, Andrew Taylor Still, insisted that fluid (particularly cerebrospinal fluid) is essential to health: "He who is able to reason will see that this great river of life must be tapped and the withering field irrigated at once, or the harvest of health be forever lost."[78] In a sense, the ultimate purpose of Craniosacral Therapy is to facilitate a return to fluid aliveness where it has been impeded.

Sutherland's Legacy

With his background in Osteopathy, Sutherland was trained to orient to the motion of bones and other structures. Sutherland's quest began as a young osteopathic student viewing a disarticulated cranium, as mentioned previously. Observing the edges of the temporal and sphenoid bones, he heard the words in his head, "beveled, like the gills of a fish, indicating articular mobility for a respiratory mechanism."[79] He considered this a "crazy thought," having learned, like other medical students, that the cranial bones were fused and did not move. The thought haunted him, however. His need to know what purpose these bevels served eventually led him to discover a breathlike phenomenon manifested in the body as rhythmical fluctuations within living fluids and tissues. He recognized a "Primary Respiration" functioning long before the lungs begin their work at birth.

When Sutherland first began perceiving Primary Respiration, he investigated it as a mechanism for "involuntary" motion in the body. Here, "involuntary" indicates that these motions are driven by an inherent life force, which he termed *potency.* These subtle motions could not be voluntarily initiated or controlled. Sutherland initially described the motion he perceived in biomechanical terms he was familiar with, such as flexion and extension, internal and external rotation. Later, as he deepened into relationship with the Breath of Life, his language changed. Where flexion/extension describes the movement of structures in relationship to each other, such as the sphenoid moving in relationship to the occiput at the spheno-basilar junction, he began to understand that the Breath of Life was more holistic and energetic. Rather than Primary Respiration being about flexion and extension of various structures, it involved primary "inhalation" and "exhalation" throughout the body, as the breathing of a unified fluid field.

"Primary" refers to the presence of this inherent breath of life prior to the "secondary" breath of air, beginning at birth.

Sensing subtle rhythmical pulsations of fluid within the body through his "thinking-feeling-seeing-knowing fingers,"[80] Sutherland understood that the CSF in the ventricles of the brain picked up the potency, or life energy, of the Breath of Life. He perceived what he termed a "transmutation" (change of state) of the Breath of Life into this inherent life force, or potency, that organizes our formation. The CSF then carries this potency to every tissue and cell in our bodies, bringing life and health. I think of potency as carrying potential, or reminding the tissues of their original potential, which may have been occluded by the conditions and traumas of life.

Prior to Sutherland, Still had already detected the importance of the CSF for health. As noted earlier, Still recognized that "the cerebrospinal fluid is one of the highest known elements that are contained in the body, and unless the brain furnishes the fluid in abundance, a disabled condition of the body will remain."[81] Sutherland expanded on this, perceiving within the CSF what he called "liquid light," or potency. He sensed this potency as doing the work of the Breath of Life within the physical body.

As Sutherland explored the cranial system, expanding far beyond the bones and membranes he began with as an osteopath, he espoused the importance of fluid (particularly CSF), and the potency within it, for health. He wrote:

> I consider the fluctuation of the cerebrospinal fluid to be the fundamental principle in the cranial concept. The "sap in the tree" is something that contains the Breath of Life, not the breath of air—something invisible. Dr. Still referred to it as one of the highest known elements in the human body, replenished from time to time. Do you think we will ever know from whence it cometh? Probably not. But it is there. That is all we need to know ... In addition there is a deeper layer of activity that has barely been touched upon. This deeper layer has to do with the energies that integrate the animated, living, homeostatic body. The day will come when they too will be catalogued and their laws understood.[82]

Sutherland came to recognize that this deeper layer of activity, the Breath of Life, mysterious and inexplicable, was manifest in all life, generating the rhythmical phenomenon he called "primary respiration," the topic of this chapter. This subtle, reciprocal expansion and contraction of the whole, preceding the secondary respiration beginning with the first breath at birth, manifests as tides moving through the entire body and beyond.

Toward the latter part of his life, Sutherland became less active in his treatments. Within the stillness, he perceived and increasingly trusted the mysterious force or bio-energy at work. He advised his students:

> Visualize a potency, an intelligent potency, that is more intelligent than your own human mentality ... You will have observed its potency and also its Intelligence, spelled with a capital I. It is something you can depend upon to do the work for you. In other words, don't try to drive the mechanism through any external force. Rely upon the Tide.[83]

The practices in presence and in settling the relational field in the previous chapters are in service of perceiving and supporting this effective activity of the potency of the Breath of Life. I like to think of myself as a vehicle for the Breath of Life. I intend to get out of the way, being as pure and present a vehicle as possible, allowing the Breath of Life to work through me. This is supported by resting in a state of being, in relative stillness, rather than a self state attached to outcomes and appearances.

Manifestations of the Breath of Life

As was already mentioned, the Breath of Life as a sacred presence generates an ordering principle Sutherland called Primary Respiration. Sutherland perceived a process of "transmutation" (change in state) of the Breath of Life, as Primary Respiration generates potency, an embodied life force, within the fluids. As Craniosacral Therapy teacher Michael Kern writes in his book, *Wisdom in the Body*, "The subtle rhythms of the Breath of Life are essentially expressions of wellness, carrying our original matrix of health into the body."[84]

In my work with clients, I have a sense of an energetic phenomenon lighting up the system. I am reminded of images of God as an old man blowing life into the clay of our bodies. My sense is not of such a personified deity, but of an infinite presence, characterized by what I can only call love. As it breathes into the field of the client, I sense an illumination, light particles sparkling through the field, infusing into the fluid, awakening the physical realm of cells and tissues. At each level, specific phenomena are apparent. Often, upon first contacting the client's body, only the denser, more physical phenomena present. As we settle and deepen together, subtler aspects of the system become apparent. We recognize these differences as relating to different levels of perception, introduced in this chapter.

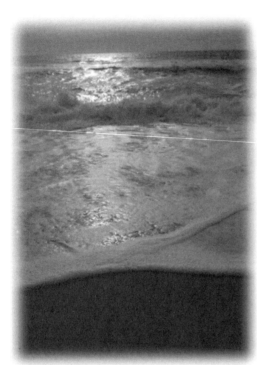

CRANIAL RHYTHMIC IMPULSE (CRI)
unstable surface waveforms, expression of unresolved
history and conditions, not a tide
6–14 cycles/min.

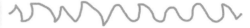

MID-TIDE/FLUID TIDE
relatively stable tide, expression of embodied life forces,
potency, with organizational, protective and healing
functions 1–3 cycles/min.

LONG TIDE
totally stable, supportive ground of primary respiration
100 second cycle:
50 sec. inhalation/50 sec. exhalation

GROUNDSWELL
Slow impulse generated by the Breath of Life from which
specific expressions of primary respiration arise, mediates
interconnection and mutuality

DYNAMIC STILLNESS
ground of stillness from which tides arise

FIGURE 21: Primary Respiration

We might compare these levels to phenomena in the ocean. When we first encounter the ocean, we are aware of the waves on its surface. These are very variable, responding to atmospheric conditions, winds, and so forth. Floating on the surface, we may easily feel rocked about and become seasick. These fluctuations relate to the various motions we may sense when first making contact with a client in cranial work. We may feel rocking, pulsations, swishing, side-to-side (lateral) fluctuations, and many different patterns of motion. We also may sense a relatively fast rhythm, like the waves on top of the sea. In Craniosacral Biodynamics, we refer to these surface waveforms relating to the conditions of the client's life as the cranial rhythmic impulse (CRI). We will begin our exploration of the levels of the perceptual ocean with these surface waves, and then look deeper.

Waves on the Surface: The Cranial Rhythmic Impulse and the Physical Body

Sutherland's initial explorations into the movements of the cranial bones, then the membranes, and other body tissues and fluids relate to this wave level of motion. Perceiving at this level involves relatively localized awareness. Within this level of awareness we may perceive patterns related to unresolved life experience and the relatively rapid rhythm of the CRI. For example, an old leg injury may present as local fluctuations or inhibited motion around the site of the injury. Rhythms of these surface wave motions, commonly eight to fourteen cycles per minute, can vary, explaining why research in Craniosacral Therapy has noted several different rates for the "cranial rhythm." This may depend on the experience level of the practitioner and methods of measurement, as examples of conditional influences.[85] These are quite different from the more stable rhythms of the tides generated by the Breath of Life and its potency, to be discussed more shortly.

The physical body is the densest, most obvious expression of life. When we initially make contact with a client, we usually sense the physical first. If I put my hands on someone's feet, I often sense the skin first. I may sense the warmth of the physical body. I may feel a pulse relating to the circulatory system and a motion relating to the person's breathing. Often, I feel rapid pulsations relating to nervous system activation, as well as a sense of density and hardness, relating to various life stresses. On a subtler level, there may be a sense of waves or fluctuations moving in various directions, perhaps even pulling toward a particular point under my hands. These patterns are expressions within the cellular tissue field of the physical body as affected by events and conditions of life.

In his early explorations, Sutherland noted patterns of motion or impeded motion between the cranial bones. In that Osteopathy is primarily oriented to the ease of mobility of bones, this was a natural place for him to start his journey. Patterns can result from early experiences in life, like being stuck in the birth canal or pulled out by forceps, as well as from later events. These include falls, knocks on the head, car accidents, or physiological traumas like cerebral vascular accident (stroke), brain tumor, or the effects of drugs, alcohol, or even genetic expression.

While a pattern of density or holding at the CRI level can have effects elsewhere in the body, they tend to be local phenomena. Their effects elsewhere can be explained through biomechanical principles. For example, an injury to the occiput puts pressure against the sphenoid bone, altering and inhibiting its motion. It may also press against nerves and blood vessels passing through the foramen magnum and jugular foramina, affecting function in regions supplied by those nerves and blood vessels. It may cause tension in the dural membranes, which is translated into tension in other parts of the connective tissue network through their tensegrity relationships.

(*Tensegrity,* a term from Buckminster Fuller, combines the words *tension* and *integrity.* It refers to structural integrity dependent on balanced tension of parts not necessarily in contact with each other, like bones held in place by soft tendons, ligaments, etc.) Here, local issues affect other local regions, as can been seen in figure 22. In this drawing, the woman has an injury in the right hip/sacroiliac area. The tension there pulls on the tensile field of the body, a tensegrity structure. The pull can be felt down the right leg and in other parts of the body.

At the CRI level of perception, we sense and can therapeutically address different areas as separate, local events, like individual waves. As we deepen into the ocean, however, we enter realms where local conditions are less significant than underlying forces creating them. For example, at these deeper levels of perception, we become aware of the unresolved forces creating the lines of tension seen in figure 22. (More to come on this in chapter 5 on the inherent treatment plan.)

In session work, we often find the client's system initially expressing the relatively rapid rhythm of the CRI and local patterning in the tissues. As we settle deeper together, often the hard, dense areas begin to feel softer and the fluctuations become slower as the wave motions settle. We frequently then begin to sense more of a holistic, tidal phenomenon, as we deepen into the ocean of life. Sills refers to this change as the "holistic shift."[86] This will be discussed in more detail in the next chapter, along with other phenomena common at the mid- or long-tide levels of perception.

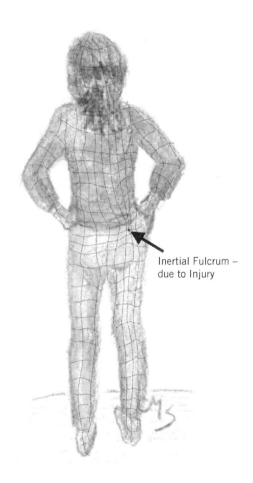

Inertial Fulcrum –
due to Injury

FIGURE 22: Tensegrity Relationships
Affected by Injury

CRI Settling Exploration

If you would like to experience settling under the CRI firsthand, please take a few minutes now to investigate with me. You may want to record these instructions and play them back to yourself to support a deeper meditative experience. (A recording is available at www.birthingyourlife.org/the-breath-of-life-book/.)

As in our previous explorations, allow yourself to find a comfortable sitting position, noting the sensations that guide you in this process. What tells you that you are comfortable or that you need to adjust something to be more comfortable? Once you are sitting quietly, place your hands on your thighs and notice how you know how firmly or lightly to place them. These sensations all provide important information. Take a moment with your hands on your thighs to notice the sensations there. How warm or cool do your thighs feel? Do they both feel the same or different? How hard or soft do they feel? Is there a sense of motion— pulsations, bubbling, or wavelike movement? Perhaps there is a sense of stillness under your hands. If so, how full or empty does this stillness seem to you? Is there a sense of presence in your thighs? How is your breath as you are inquiring into the sense of contact at your thighs? Can you sense your breath as well as where your hands are? How much of the whole presents itself to you?

All of these are sensations we may sense when first making contact with a client's body. If there is a sense of motion, note the direction of the motion. Is it all moving in the same direction? Which way? Does it seem chaotic, with one part moving in one direction and another part in a different direction? How fast or slow is this motion?

Allow yourself to be curious about what you sense. Can you be present with it, just observing? Or is there a sense of worry, such as "Oh, no, my left and right sides are different!" Or is there a need to fix what doesn't seem right? How do you sense something as right or not? Do you have a sense of patterning or shapes under your hands?

After listening for a few minutes, do you notice any changes? How is your breath now? Is it different in any way than it was earlier? As you continue to listen, what speaks to you of settling, quieting, relaxing? What changes in your perception as you intend to orient to settling? To enhance your sense of settling, you may want to try slowing down your breath. Let yourself really feel the support of the surface under you. Can you rest into it a bit more? Remember your list of resources. What can support you just now in settling just a bit more? Does anything change as you support yourself in settling deeper?

When you feel like you have explored enough for now, gently open your eyes if they have been closed and orient to the space around you before you continue reading. You may want to take some notes about what you experienced.

Deepening into the Ocean: Fluid Tide

Settling with my hands on my client's feet, we deepen together. As the little storms and breezes of patterning and activation begin to soften, we both experience a sense of smoothness, a wholeness, as the holistic shift emerges. The motion I sense then shifts. At first subtle, then gradually becoming stronger, I detect a sense of energy building. Continuing to deepen into stillness, widening my perception, and orienting to the client's midline, I sense a percolating, which seems to be bubbling at the base of the spine. I am reminded of the lumbosacral waterbed or cistern, a lake of CSF between the L2 and S2 vertebrae where we often sense a building of potency. This life energy seems to be transmuted to the CSF right there in that lake.

As the energy builds, it begins to surge up the midline. At the same time, I sense the whole field of tissues and fluids widening out from the midline, filling as potency feeds every cell of the body. I recognize this midline-oriented motion as inhalation of the fluid tide. It lasts twelve to fifteen seconds, then pauses, as if resting in the stillness from whence it arose, before receding back down and in toward midline in exhalation, returning to source. I find myself holding a whole fluid field, like a sphere of fluid, larger than the client's physical body, which seems to be suspended within it. I am reminded of the embryo and suddenly feel as if I am holding one in my hands. My heart opens as I sense a little one growing and pulsating within its fluid sac. A little one with its translucent tissues barely distinguished around its vibrant midline. A little one that is mostly midline, suspended in its amniotic fluid, just being, just growing. I feel protective and at the same time amazed at the biointelligence at work here, growing, differentiating. I sense a fluid bundle of brilliant life energy coming into embodied form.

I feel honored and touched to witness this mysterious unfolding of life energy, clearly directed by the potency of the Breath of Life. Within this wholistic, embryonic fluid field, I sense areas of holding, where the fluid tide does not express as fully and easily. As I continue to listen and witness, I sense the potency gathering at one of these points, as the fluid fluctuates and deviates around it. I observe the unfolding of a highly intelligent healing process, the inherent treatment plan being expressed. The client's system drops into stillness as the formative forces affecting this chosen fulcrum settle into a state of balance. With my hands in contact with this area, I sense energy being discharged from it in the form of heat, pulsations, and buzzing.

Then there is a deeper settling, and I have a feeling of the entire organism reorganizing itself now that this fulcrum is no longer an organizing point within it. I find myself sensing the heart forming as the embryo folds, little arm and leg buds appearing. I watch the show as energies move here and there, fluids and tissues shift, and then a new order emerges as the fluid tide resumes, with a stronger push, or drive, than before. I am again in awe of the workings of what William Sutherland called "Intelligence with a capital I"— an intrinsic and mysterious wisdom emerging from invisible depths.

Staying with the ocean metaphor and submerging ourselves in the ocean waters, we discover motion related to a deeper tide. This is smoother and slower than the surface waves, while still somewhat affected by individual conditions and experience. In Craniosacral Biodynamics we call this the mid-tide or fluid tide. Fluid tide is a classical cranial osteopathic term referring to the manifestation of Primary Respiration within the fluids of the body. *Mid-tide* is a term coined by Sills to expand this concept to include a more wholistic orientation. It incorporates the life force or potency that manifests in the fluids, generating fluid tide, and organizes cells and tissues into form,

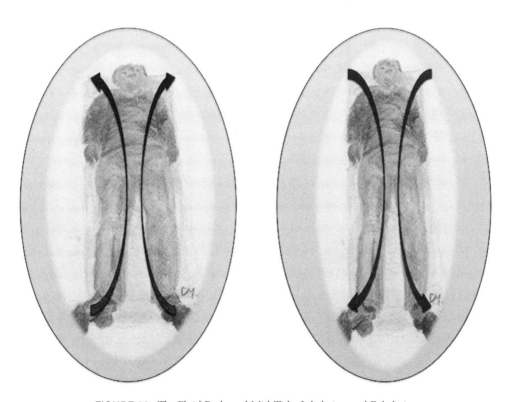

FIGURE 23 : The Fluid Body and Mid-Tide: Inhalation and Exhalation

as well as generating their rhythmical motion, called motility. Mid-tide refers to the expression of Primary Respiration within the entire body, including fluids, tissues, and the potent bioenergetic field Becker termed "the biosphere," which we sense extending twenty inches or fifty centimeters beyond the surface of the skin.

Mid-tide, and the fluid body it expresses within, is an embodied expression of Primary Respiration. The rhythm of its breath is slower than the CRI, faster than long tide, and also has a very different feel from these. More tangible and liquid than the tidal body, the fluid body includes the physical fluids of the physical body (blood, lymph, intercellular fluids, CSF, interstitial fluids, etc.). The fluid body is sensed as one united field of action, all filling and emptying at the same time, in contrast to the more localized CRI level of perception.

Deepening into a mid-tide level of perception takes us into a sense of wholeness. We begin to sense motion of the whole body in relation to a midline running vertically through the center, a long fulcrum of stillness centering the motion around it. The midline of our fluid wholeness, which we call the fluid body or field, relates to space within the spinal canal within the spinal cord, or the neural tube of the embryo. This tube is both filled with and suspended within cerebrospinal fluid. Every cell of every structure in the physical body moves or is moved with inhalation and exhalation of the mid-tide. Rather than the mobility of bones moving in relation to each other, at this fluid level of perception, the motility, or intrinsic motion within each structure, becomes apparent and significant. We sense a reciprocal fluctuation, like filling and receding of every cell with the inhalation and exhalation of mid-tide. Every tissue, including, for example, each cranial bone, is filling along with every other structure of the body. We perceive the true fluidity of each part.

Remember that we are composed predominantly of fluid. Even bones, the densest structures in our physical bodies, are made up mainly of fluid. Unless restricted by an inertial holding pattern, every bone and structure is breathing together with the mid-tide. The wholeness we perceive within the fluid body is not about how one structure affects another, as with the CRI-level of perception. Here, we are perceiving a unified tensile field breathing with the Breath of Life. Sills writes, "Motility is an expression of potency as an inner breath in every cell. When you perceive motility at a mid-tide level, each tissue structure is sensed to be part of a unified cellular-fluid field and the quality of motion sensed is fluidic and holistic."[87]

This deeper tidal motion, generated by potency, is an aspect of Primary Respiration. Like the breath of air in the lungs, it inhales and exhales, but much more slowly. With two to three cycles per minute, we may sense a surge rising up the midline as the entire body seems to fill, widening and expanding with inhalation, as potency potentially infuses every cell in the body. In exhalation, there is a sense of receding, narrowing, returning to midline, and settling back down into the earth or toward the feet. As we become more familiar with this mid-tide phenomenon, we may begin to sense its inhalation and exhalation involving an energetic field, the biosphere mentioned previously, extending out around the physical body. This fluid body includes all the fluids of the physical body along with their bioenergetic field, extending out twenty inches or fifty centimeters around the physical body. While the fluid body and mid-tide, being deeper in the ocean, are less affected by the conditions of life, they are responsive to life events. Potency acts to organize, protect, and heal in relation to both biodynamic and additional conditional forces. We will learn more about this process in the next chapter.

Deepening further into the ocean, we perceive a tide slower and more stable still than the mid-tide. At the long-tide level of perception, we experience a seemingly infinite field of light, unaffected by the history and conditions of one's life.

Before moving onto look at long tide, let's take a little time to explore the possibility of sensing mid-tide.

Mid-Tide Exploration

Here is a perceptual exercise that you may find helpful. Please don't worry if you don't sense mid-tide this first time. It can take practice to perceive such subtle phenomena. This is just a beginning!

Let's return to sitting comfortably, including noticing the sensations that help you to find that position. Again, you may want to record these instructions and play them back to yourself to enable you to have your eyes closed and be more inwardly focused. (A recording is available at www.birthingyourlife.org/the-breath-of-life-book.) Once you are comfortable, take a little time to attend to your breath, checking where and how you sense it, the quality of your breath, how fast or slow it is, how it is to be with, and how easy or effortful it is. Can you begin to rest in your breath? Can you sense the places where your body is making contact with what you are sitting on? Can you feel your hands making contact with whatever they are in contact with? You may want to rest them on your thighs to facilitate sensing what is happening in your own body, through your hands.

As in our CRI settling exploration, let yourself become aware of any sense of motion or stillness in your body. This may be through your hands, or you may sense it more internally. What is your sense of motion in your body? Are there pulsations, waves, to-ings, and fro-ings? How fast or slow are these motions? Are there patterns you are aware of? Whatever you notice, allow yourself to acknowledge these sensations and intend to settle under them. Listen for any sense of something slower, softer, smoother. What speaks to you of settling, relaxing, resting? You may begin to sense your breathing become slower, your tissues feeling softer, the motion you are aware of becoming quieter and slower. Remind yourself of resource to help yourself settle.

As we begin to deepen, let's practice orienting to mid-tide and the fluid body. Allow yourself to become aware of anything that speaks to you of fluidity in your body. Again, this may be a sense of softening, as tissues begin to melt and become more fluid. There may be a sense of motions slowing down and becoming more coherent. Is there any sense of motion toward or away from a vertical centerline of your body? To begin to become aware of midline, it can be helpful to first inquire into your sense of your spine. This is a boney midline within your body, running from the tip of your tailbone all the way up through your neck. Do you have a sense of that as midline? If you sense motion, you may notice that the midline is relatively still. It serves as a fulcrum of stillness, in the center of tidal motion.

In settling further into fluid body and midline, there may be more of a sense of wholeness, sensing more of the whole of your body, rather than separate parts. You may begin to have a sense of a subtle filling of your whole body. In the inhalation phase of mid-tide, there may be a sense of building, surging up midline, filling, widening out from midline. This is followed by a sense of emptying or receding in exhalation, narrowing back or returning in toward midline, dropping down toward the tail. Each phase lasts twelve to fifteen seconds. You may sense a pause at the end of a phase, as the system rests briefly into stillness. Allowing yourself to be curious about this mid-tide rhythm, two to three cycles per minute, can you rest in awareness of the whole of you? Rather than searching for anything, let the perceptions come to you as you settle back and down into the earth, into whatever supports you. With a wide field of perception, resting in midline in the center, allow your senses to inform you.

Gently widening your view, you may become aware of a sense of a fluid field extending out beyond the boundaries of your skin about twenty inches or fifty centimeters. Can you allow yourself to rest in a sense of your physical body being suspended and supported within this larger field?

Don't worry if these perceptions are not immediately obvious to you. It takes time to learn to perceive in this way. Can you allow yourself to rest in curiosity, wondering how these phenomena will present to you?

When you feel like you have rested in this perceptual state for long enough, gently bring your awareness back to your physical body, the places where it makes contact with what you are sitting on, your breath, and other sensations. Gently open your eyes if they have been closed and look around the room you are in to orient yourself. You may want to take some notes about your experience. I recommend practicing this meditation frequently to develop your ability to sense at this level of perception. I suspect you will notice changes occurring over time as your perceptual skills develop, and as your system is able to settle more deeply with the meditation.

It is common to sense the mid-tide and fluid body as the system begins to settle under CRI. As it settles further, it is not unusual to sense a deeper level of the ocean. The next section introduces long tide.

Deepening into a Field of Radiance: The Long Tide

Resting in stillness, I sense a deepening in my client. Actually, we share the deepening. Our separation as individuals seems less relevant. Together, we inhabit a field of radiance. Quiet, slow, powerful. I feel my attention guided by the fiery, airy nature of long-tide as it streams in from somewhere beyond the realms of definition. It seems to pour in toward the client's midline as if from beyond the horizon, lighting it up. My senses seem to shift into a more visual mode, as I see/feel the light. This streaming of exhalation at the long-tide level seems to go on forever, but has actually been measured as a consistent fifty seconds. There is a pause, a deepening into stillness, and then the streaming resumes, this time emerging from the brilliant midline, expanding in the ever-growing spaciousness, out toward the horizon, the mysterious source from whence it came. I sense my awareness expanding further, carried by the long tide.

Within the client's system, I am aware of the light doing its work, sometimes very quickly, like wind or fire striking its object. This field of radiance of the long-tide, or tidal body, feels more airy to me than fluid, although I can sense the fluid body, a more embodied expression of Primary Respiration, suspended within it. What I feel most strongly is a sense of peace and awe. This is the Breath of Life in action. I can almost touch the love in its rawest form. There is nothing for me to do here. I rest. I appreciate. I receive. I love. I listen. I dissolve.

The long tide is sensed in Craniosacral Biodynamics as a very slow, extremely subtle tidal rhythm streaming out beyond the physical body toward the horizon in all directions and back in toward midline at a constant rate of fifty seconds out and fifty seconds in, or one hundred for a complete cycle. Becker wrote of his discovery of this very slow tide he called the *large tide:* "It's obviously always been there, but it was startling at first. I had been working for about fifteen or twenty minutes on somebody, and all of a sudden, I was aware of the fact that it felt like the whole patient was expanding. It was like watching fingers of the tide coming in, seeping through the tissues." Unable to work out where it comes from or disappears to, he further writes, "I think we're in simple rhythm with the farthest stars, ten times a minute by way of the cerebrospinal fluid and a minute and a half apart for this large tide." The "ten times a minute" tide relates to what we call the CRI, which Becker notes is easier to explain because of its fluid, contained nature. This larger long tide is consistently one hundred seconds long, about a minute and a half, and seems to be boundless.[88]

Perceiving the long tide is often associated with a sense of light or radiance. It can feel quite airy and ethereal, even spiritual. The long tide streams through the body but is not limited to the physical body. It seems to be the first stepping down of the Breath of Life into what we call the Tidal Body. This consists of a field of life force generated

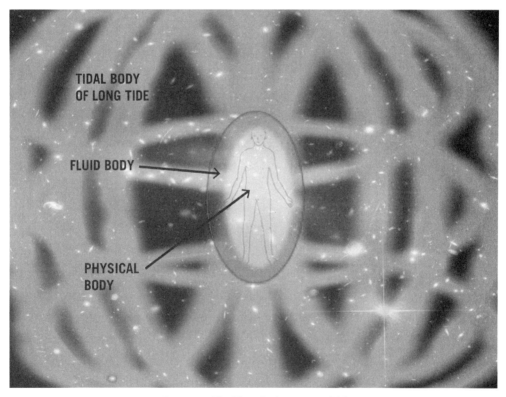

FIGURE 24: The Three Bodies in Long Tide
Background is MACS J0416, Credit: NASA, ESA, CXC, NRAO/AUI/NSF, STScI, and G. Ogrean (Stanford University), Acknowledgment: NASA, ESA, J. Lotz (STScI), and the HFF team; http://hubblesite.org/image/3713/gallery

by the Breath of Life, manifesting locally as a bioelectric ordering field related to the individual. (More on this in chapter 6.)

We can sense the long tide as moving through a field of radiance organized in relation to a midline of light. When perceiving long tide, I often have a sense of a sparkliness streaming in toward the central midline, which seems to light up as the sparkles arrive from their mysterious source. As mentioned above, this very slow, subtle tide seems to expand out toward the horizon in all directions, as if enlarging forever, and returning from beyond the horizon as if from nowhere, each cycle inhaling for fifty seconds and exhaling for fifty seconds. This stable rhythm is unaffected by life conditions and found universally in nature. For example, Seifritz, a scientist who in the 1950s studied slime mold—a simple unicellular organism consisting of protoplasm and many nuclei—and discovered a constant streaming through the slime mold at a stable rate, reversing direction every fifty seconds. Seifritz stated, "Could we but understand the cause of this constant movement, we would be nearer to an understanding of what life is." He noted that, when he applied various toxins to the slime mold, it appeared to shrivel and the motion seemed to stop for a time. When it started again, however, it acted as if it had been in motion the whole time, as if it had never been interrupted, indicating an ongoing rhythm, more basic or primary than the visible flow. He declared, "We must be very close indeed to the question, what is life?"[89] The stable one-hundred-second rhythm he observed seems to be relevant to all phenomena in nature, supporting our perception that it is an organizing principle for all natural phenomena. There was even a recent one-hundred-second recording representing the sound of the big bang.[90]

Long-Tide Exploration

In exploring our sense of long tide, we may find ourselves deepening gradually, like dropping deeper into the ocean or taking an elevator down several floors. The elevator doors may open as we pass through the CRI and then mid-tide levels of perception.

Again, you may want to record these instructions and play them back to yourself to enable you to settle more deeply and focus more internally in this exploration. (A recording is available at www.birthingyourlife.org/the-breath-of-life-book.)

Take some time to settle again into a comfortable seated position, noting the sensations that guide you in this process, as well as the qualities of your breath and how your body rests into the support of gravity under you. Notice any sense of CRI, of surface waves, to-ings and fro-ings, pulsations, or other faster motions or patterns that present. Allow yourself to acknowledge these and intend to settle deeper, listening for a sense of wholeness and Primary Respiration. As you deepen, you may find yourself sensing the fluidity of mid-tide we have visited previously. This may include a sense of wholeness, midline, building, surging up midline, filling, widening out from midline in inhalation, and narrowing back toward midline and down toward the tail or feet with the sense of emptying or receding in exhalation. Allow yourself to rest in whatever sense of mid-tide you may be experiencing. Again, this is not about looking for anything in particular, but intending to deepen, widen your field of perception, resting. I often think of perception in Craniosacral Biodynamics as being like a movie screen upon which images are projected, rather than actively searching for anything.

After taking some time to settle with whatever you are sensing, allow yourself to widen your field of awareness even further. Without losing your sense of midline, allow your awareness to begin to widen out beyond your physical body, beyond the fluid field extending twenty inches or fifty centimeters out, widening further out to fill the whole room. If this is comfortable for you, let your awareness widen further, out toward the horizon in all directions, however far you can extend it without losing a sense of your central midline and ground. This is not about spacing out but rather about widening your field of perception, which usually takes some practice.

Resting in this wide field, you may begin to find your awareness being carried in toward your midline or out toward the horizon very, very slowly. Long tide takes fifty seconds to complete an exhalation or inhalation. Within this very slow rhythm, there may be a sense of faster, windlike swirling or spiraling. There may be a sense of sparkly, radiant light. Often there is a sense of being suspended in a very, very wide field of support. How is it to rest into this wide field?

Allowing yourself to rest here, notice what arises for you. It may be an expansive, blissful experience, but there may be other, more conditioned experiences also associated with this kind of spaciousness and support.

After some time of resting within this wide field, let your awareness return to a sense of fluid body, the fluid field closer to your physical body, perhaps touching in again with a sense of mid-tide.

Within that fluid field, you also find your physical body. Coming back to sense of breath and the support of the earth and her gravity under you, is there any sense for you of your physical body being suspended within or supported by the fluid, and the fluid body in turn being suspended within the field of long tide? Over time, you can develop an ability to be with all three bodies or fields, accessing fields within fields of support.

When you are ready, gently bring your awareness back to the room you are in, looking around to orient yourself. You may want to make some time to make some notes about your experience to refer back to later.

These meditations can be very helpful in developing perceptual skills for session work with clients. As we continue to listen and deepen with our clients, we often sense a pausing of the tides or even a sense of dissolving of all motion and form. At the bottom of the ocean, like in deepest outer space, we encounter stillness. If you have seen films of deep sea diving, you begin to get the picture of this deepening process. Becker described an "alive and dynamic stillness," from which Sills derived the shorter term *dynamic stillness*.[91] Unrelated to our personal conditions of life, it is in stillness that the deepest healing can occur. As we shall see, in Craniosacral Biodynamics we aim to settle under the CRI waves, to rest in stillness, and to allow the deeper tides and potency to express as needed.

Returning to Source: Dynamic Stillness

Resting with my client's system softly suspended in my liquid, spacious hands, I sense a deepening. Something in me lets go, as seems also true within the client. We deepen together into dynamic stillness. There is nothing to do here. There is no sense of motion, but there is a powerful aliveness, a vibrant potency. My hands no longer seem important. My client and I are one within this stillness. We are suspended within a powerful intelligence, the source of health, the ground of all being. I feel as if we float together within an endless field of light, of space beyond space, beyond time, beyond story and history. As we rest here, I recognize the bubbling of potency, life energy welling up from a deep, invisible cavern. Sparks of light seem to emit from this depth of stillness. When we emerge, I notice the client's system seems different. Various patterns and their organizing fulcrums have disappeared, apparently resolved by what Becker called the Silent Partner.[92] *My job is to be still, recognize and respect the stillness, resonate with it, deepen into it, support its work with my intention to be its partner. I feel deeply honored in this process. I choose to be a vehicle for the Breath of Life to do its work. I surrender.*

Dynamic stillness is the ground of being from which life and form emerge. We may experience it at various times during session work. As practitioners, we aim to rest our awareness in stillness, and to perceive from there. It is always present, although it may be occluded by the patterns and effects of history, including various traumas one has had to adapt to in life. We can, however, choose to orient to it, deepening beyond the surface waves of history, and even deeper and wider than the tides. Orienting to the stillness can support the client's system in remembering that it too can access this immense resource.

Becker describes stillness as "the Silent Partner." In reading his attempts to describe it, we can appreciate how beyond description and words it is:

> Actually it boils down to what do you surrender to now? Your Silent Partner is a fulcrum point; it's absolutely still. There's no energy in motion in the Silent Partner, none. It's all energy, but it's not in motion. Actually it is the source of energy, the state from which energy comes. It isn't energy in motion, it's just pure potency. It's omnipotent. There is no motion, and yet it's all motion. It just is, and you surrender to it … It's a living stillness that our conscious awareness can be aware of. This conscious awareness is with our big Mind, not our little mind. Awareness is the acceptance of something.[93]

It is helpful to remember that the states, tides, and phenomena we describe in Craniosacral Biodynamics are efforts to put into words profound, wordless perceptual experiences. When we touch the mystery, words may be relatively useless or irrelevant. We do, however, feel moved to share this amazing experience with others, particularly if we want to facilitate them learning to perceive it themselves. When we perceive, the experience, no matter how subtle and beyond the ordinary, is very real and present. Dynamic stillness may be ineffable, but it soaks us, nourishes us, bathes us in unmistakable ways when we orient to its presence. Becker writes:

> While this may sound esoteric, it is a tangible experience. Once in a while when I'm treating patients in my office, you can take the stillness in that room, cut it with a knife, and make an igloo out of it—it gets that quiet. What brings it on? I haven't any idea, and who cares? It is there to meet the need for something that is going on for that particular individual. Where it comes from and where it disappears to is not important. It's a way of life, a way of Life with a capital L.[94]

Dynamic stillness as a ground from which the Breath of Life and life itself emerge into form is reminiscent of physicist David Bohm's "implicate order," from which we unfold our experience:

> In the enfolded [or implicate] order, space and time are no longer the dominant factors determining the relationships of dependence or independence of different elements. Rather, an entirely different sort of basic connection of elements is possible, from which our ordinary notions of space and time, along with those of separately existent material particles, are abstracted as forms derived from the deeper order. These ordinary

notions in fact appear in what is called the "explicate" or "unfolded" order, which is a special and distinguished form contained within the general totality of all the implicate orders.[95]

When we slow ourselves down, deepening into the underlying stillness, we perceive our source, being prior to form, our enfolded potential prior to and beyond our unfolded shape and structure. This state of being is referred to in various spiritual traditions, such as the emptiness of Chan or Zen Buddhism. For example, Zen Master Hongzhi wrote:

> Vast and far-reaching without boundary, secluded and pure, manifesting light, this spirit is without obstruction. Its brightness does not shine out but can be called empty and inherently radiant. Its brightness, inherently purifying, transcends causal conditions beyond subject and object. Subtle but preserved, illumined and vast, also it cannot be spoken of as being or nonbeing, or discussed with images or calculations. Right in here the central pivot turns, the gateway opens. You accord without laboring and accomplish without hindrance.[96]

In Craniosacral Biodynamics we speak of returning to the "original matrix," where what I see as our original potential remains accessible and untouched, regardless of how life has treated us. Stillness awaits us, beyond and beneath the busy-ness and doing-ness of everyday life. Although practiced meditators can learn to carry a sense of stillness with them into their "fetch wood, carry water" activities, it is not easy to access stillness in our generally sped-up, activated states of modern life. It is there, however, waiting patiently for our return. Here, I think of my mother, who was always such a "doer" during her life. In the last phase of her life, as dementia deepened and her body refused to move much, I witnessed her disappearing into a mysterious realm beyond the ordinary. She seemed at times, for almost the first time in her life, to experience peace. My sense was that she stopped struggling, stopped trying to do, and surrendered, just as Becker advised us to do in relation to the Silent Partner, although perhaps for different reasons. Similarly, I had an octogenarian client many years ago who considered her occupation to be preparing for death. She loved receiving Craniosacral Therapy. Together, we would deepen into stillness, where she would experience a deeply restful, peaceful state uncommon in her life. I remember her commenting as she emerged from this state, "Ah, this is what it will be like!"

Hopefully, we don't need to wait until death to return to the stillness from which we emerge. In Craniosacral Biodynamics, stillness is the heart and ground of healing.

Whatever other processes we perceive, stillness underlies them. We may encounter the stillness as a deep dropping or settling during the session. We may also encounter "gateways to stillness" at the end of an inhalation or exhalation phase of the mid-tide, or within the spacious expansiveness of the long tide. Other still points may also occur during our sessions, as the system pauses or deepens, entering a state of balance of different forces, where the various fluctuations and shifting of potency seem to settle and still, if even for a moment. Similarly, when the inherent treatment plan unfolds at a mid-tide level, the tide often seems to stop while the potency works with a particular inertial issue. It usually starts up again when the work is done, indicating integration and completion of a process. It is as if this ever-present stillness is always there in the background. When the activities of life process settle and calm enough, we sense its presence and can rest into its support. Of course, the option of orienting to stillness is always available.

Sutherland's advice to "be still and know" relates to the biblical verse "Be still, and know that I *am* God: I will be exalted among the heathen, I will be exalted in the earth."[97] When the practitioner orients to stillness, while staying open to perceiving other levels of expression within the client's system, we find the work can deepen and proceed in a gentler, more resourced way. It seems there is the possibility of returning to stillness at any time, and, from there, re-emerging, perhaps (usually) somewhat "exalted" and transformed. I see this as a process of returning to our original potential, like the embryo emerging into form from the implicate order of stillness, suspended within the waters of the womb. When we return to this state, we can access the original potential still held for us by the stillness.

Dynamic Stillness Exploration

For this exploration, you may want to record the instructions and play them back to yourself to support your settling more deeply. (A recording is available at www.birthingyourlife *.org/the-breath-of-life-book.)*

As in our previous explorations, allow yourself to settle into a comfortable seated position. Take note of the sensations of comfort or discomfort guiding you in this settling. Also, note your sense of breath and how your body rests into the support of gravity under it, particularly sensing the places where your body makes contact. Notice any sense of motion or patterning arising as you intend to settle. Allow yourself to continue to settle deeper, perhaps with a sense of mid-tide or even long tide as in our previous explorations. Allow yourself to be aware of any sense of building, filling, surging up midline, widening in inhalation of mid-tide and settling, receding, narrowing in exhalation. You may become aware of a slower, deeper tide, a sense of streaming toward or away from you as you allow your aware-ness to widen out toward the horizon just as far as is comfortable without losing a sense of ground and presence. Take your time and allow yourself to rest with your perceptions, not looking for anything, just receiving what comes, with an intention to orient to the depths of the ocean, resting in fields within fields of support.

After resting in this wide field of perception for some time, allow yourself to let go of any sense of motion, even long tide. Orient to the stillness within which the tides present. You may have a sense of a pause or moment of stillness at the end of inhalation or exhalation. Allow yourself to rest into the stillness of the pause. Or you may have a sense of deepening and widening even further, beyond motion, resting in the ground of dynamic stillness. This is an alive stillness. Allow yourself to sense the aliveness of it. You may become aware of a sense of potent building, or light. Potency can build within the stillness. You may find yourself feeling like you can rest deeply, supported by unseen forces, a vast field of stillness.

Allow yourself to rest and be nourished by this field. From within the stillness, at some point, you may have a sense of motion arising again, perhaps a sense of the slow streaming of long tide, and/or the more embodied filling of mid-tide. As you sense the tides again, take note of anything that seems different from how it was before you deepened into the stillness.

When you are ready, gently bring yourself back to awareness of your physical body, which may feel as if it is suspended within fluid suspended within the field of long tide suspended within a vast field of dynamic stillness. Gently open your eyes, and look around the room to orient yourself. Take your time. Feel your feet and how your body is supported by gravity under it. Feel your breath. Move your body gently as it feels right to you. You may want to take some time to make some notes about your experience.

Emerging from Stillness into Form

Becker writes:

> When a baby is born, the first inspiration starts the breathing mechanism, the respi-ratory movements needed as we walk about on Earth. But even before the respiratory movements begin, all during the time the child is in utero, there is a rhythmic to-and-fro, ebb-and-flow, a rhythmic movement of every part of the body during the develop-ing months. I am convinced that this begins right from the time of conception.[98]

Sills describes how, at the moment of conception, the Breath of Life ignites and a field of light emerges in relation to the conceptus.[99] Within this field, a local expression of long tide emerges. The embryo begins to form within its bioelectric field, guided by the potency of the Breath of Life. This may sound like a lovely fantasy, but its reality seems to exist beyond our perceptual experience as biodynamic practitioners (or other energy/bodyworkers). What we call the quantum midline, at the center of the field of light, appears to be the subject described in a revolutionary book, *The Rainbow and The Worm*.[100] Its author, scientist Mae-Wan Ho, discusses her research demonstrating that an energetic midline within unicellular wormlike creatures is responsive to their environment and apparently organizing their form.[101] She sees quantum coherence as key to our formation and biological functioning, as well as emphasizing the importance of electromagnetic fields, and the dangers of altering them, for example through the effects of mobile phones.

Our work of Craniosacral Biodynamics orients to phenomena within these subtle fields, including the ground of dynamic stillness from which it all emerges. Holding our clients supported within fields within fields of support, we often sense a dissolution of form into relative stillness, followed by an emergence of something new. We may sense a tiny embryo in our hands and the formation of a new being. The next chapter describes this process of healing through the unfolding of what we call "the inherent treatment plan" within session work.

5

Honoring Intelligence

The Inherent Treatment Plan

Let me keep my mind on what matters, which is my work, which is mostly standing still and learning to be astonished.

—MARY OLIVER, "The Messenger"[102]

*T*he journey together has begun. I stand quietly beside my client who is settling on the treatment table. We have talked for a few minutes, checking in on how she is, on what resources and supports her, and what issues or intentions she has arrived at the session with today. I have guided her in settling into a sense of breath on the treatment table, sensing the support of the table under her and anything else that supports her. I settle myself deeper into a sense of my physical body as suspended within the larger fluid body and its mid-tide, suspended within the still wider immensity of the tidal body, the field of radiance of the long tide. I sense its radiance streaming in toward my midline, lighting it up, and streaming ever so slowly back out to its mysterious source. Continuing to deepen and widen, I sense myself at rest with my client as the vibrant field of dynamic stillness holds us in its ever-present embrace.

Widening my awareness, I now allow the client's midline to be the center of my field of perception. I am, as always, amazed that I can sense the edge of her fluid body just in front of me. Somehow, I knew where it was and stood just outside of it. I am also struck by a sense of what feels to me like burning in her midline area. I recognize this as an activation of her sympathetic nervous system with its sympathetic chain running down either side of the spine.

I take note of this, remembering she had told me about her feeling of intense stress in her life this week. Although I have become accustomed to sensing things like this from the side of the table, I still wonder at how this is possible. I am reminded of the potential resonance when two beings come into contact and the subtle energetic communication between us.

As I feel our separate systems coming into communion, I sense a settling in the fields suspended within fields where we meet. I ask her if she feels ready for some contact. She agrees. I let her know I am moving to her feet, making contact at the tops of her feet, after slowly moving to the foot of the table, and settling a bit further there. With my client's midline still the center of my field of perception, I allow my hands to softly make contact, aware that they are moving through her sensitive fluid field to do so. I check with her how the contact feels to her. She replies, "Wonderful, warm, ahhhh." I sense we are already settling into the contact and no further negotiation is needed. I suggest we continue to settle together, deepening, softening, resting.

With first contact on her feet, I am taken aback by the tension and hardness I feel there. Although this is not uncommon, I am always surprised when reminded of how we tend to tense ourselves against the world. I hold her feet with a sense of us both being suspended together within the wider fields of fluid and tidal bodies, and dynamic stillness. I sense rapid pulsations and buzzing, which I recognize as nervous system activation. As I orient to stillness, these begin to slow down and soften. I notice her feet are also softening and feeling a bit warmer, as if more inhabited. My client takes a deep breath and comments that she feels her feet more than she did before, as if they were more alive and part of her. Another wave of buzzing arises and settles as the nervous system discharges. Some fluid fluctuations draw my attention. I acknowledge their presence quietly to myself and continue to deepen and widen my awareness. Her midline is the center of my field of awareness, with her physical, fluid, and tidal bodies extending out around it.

Gradually, there is a deeper settling. I begin to sense the feet as connected to not only the legs, but also the trunk. I begin to have a sense of my client's midline lighting up and widening, coming out from behind the clouds of her conditions. I notice I feel as if my hands extend up the back of her body, up to her mid-back region. She comments that she feels her legs are really part of her now. I ask how far up her body she senses the connection. "To about my middle back, I think," she says. I appreciate again the way we can communicate energetically, the words confirming what I was sensing. As we talk, I sense more softening. I feel as if my hands are completely immersed in fluid, within the larger fields holding us. Now, they feel like they extend up to the top of her head. This is a familiar feeling for me, as it is how I often sense holistic shift, a very unique way to be sure.

I feel as if I am holding a tiny baby, her whole little body in my hands. My heart opens. I feel a warm, tender protectiveness as I would with a little one. My hands have dissolved now. We are one. Together we are suspended in the forces of life. We dance the subtle fluid dance of Craniosacral Biodynamics. I notice a sense of building, filling, surging up the midline, even though my hands are still on her feet. I feel as if I am in contact with the whole physical body, suspended within the fluid body, suspended within the field of radiance of long tide, all infused with the ground of dynamic stillness, as I sense this inhalation of the mid-tide. I note for myself that the holistic shift has deepened. Deepening further with it, I listen. There is nothing for me to do here. The inherent treatment plan has begun. I wait with curiosity as to how it will unfold.

As I wait and deepen, I begin to become aware of a pull toward her right hip. I notice the inhalation and exhalation of the mid-tide seem weaker on the right side. I get a sense of the tide, and even her whole body arching around that right hip. As I listen for what organizes this pattern, I sense a fulcrum, or organizing center, in the middle of the hip area. Well, actually, it seems to be within the right psoas. I wait, settling, widening. I don't want to focus in on this area of interest. A point in the right psoas area seems to light up as if coming forward out of the whole, although still suspended within the three-body suspensory system. I check in with my client and let her know I feel drawn to move my hands to make contact with her right hip/psoas area. She responds by saying, "Oh, I forgot to mention I've been having pain and stiffness almost every day in my right hip. How did you know?"

She loves having my hands there, one in front over the psoas, and one under her hip, as we settle in at this new point of contact. Here, I marvel at the unfolding of the inherent treatment plan. There is a sense of swirling, fluctuating fluids, as the conditional forces held in this inertial fulcrum seek balance with the potency containing them. As I orient to the stillness at the heart of the fulcrum, suspended within the surrounding supportive fields of fluid body, tidal body, and dynamic stillness, I sense a quieting, a deepening, as these forces settle into a state of balance in dynamic equilibrium. It seems as if the stillness in the fulcrum is communing with the larger ground of dynamic stillness holding us. I sense an intense heat pouring out into my hand in front, then a pulsation and sensation of sharpness. As I hold this in my awareness suspended within the fields around us, the heat gradually softens. The pulsations cease. I sense the tissues between my hands softening, spreading, and vibrating. A gentle, soothing warmth infuses the area as potency spreads through the tissues, where inertia reigned before.

I become aware of new motion in different parts of the body. The neck seems to pull to the left, the sphenoid rotates, the legs seem to move chaotically in different directions as the whole system reorganizes. Now that this inertial fulcrum has dissolved and its inertial forces dissipated, the system begins to orient more fully to the midline, remembering its original intention. I sense a powerful surge of potency up the midline as mid-tide resumes with a strong inhalation. I sense this part of the treatment plan has completed. I check in with my client, who is delighted with how soft and free her hip feels. She tells me about a memory that arose for her during the session, which she had not thought about in years. As a teen-ager, she had followed a dare to climb a tree. She had been terrified but was determined to prove to her brother that she could do it and be as good as any boy. She had managed to get to the top and was on her way down when she lost her balance and fell. She fortunately landed on some soft grass but her hip had smashed into a twig. It was the one area really hurting afterward. It had eventually stopped bothering her until just recently, and she had completely forgotten about the incident. "Do you think you just took that experience out of my hip?" she asked. I am careful to explain to her that I didn't do much of anything, but the Intelligence of her system may have just resolved what was left over from that experience. As we complete the session, I rest again into a sense of awe at the Intelligence of the "unerring potency" and its inherent treatment plan, and the power of just holding it, being with it in appreciation and respect.

As Sutherland's understanding of Primary Respiration and its effects in the body developed, his ultimate interest shifted from the outer form of the tissues to the underlying formative forces at work in his patients. He realized that the changes in his patients' conditions or the corrections of their osteopathic lesions were due to an intelligent force operating through the body fluids, rather than to his specific manipulations or corrective work. As we have seen, he named this force "potency," and understood it to be a transmutation of the Breath of Life into embodied form. Where his earlier work had oriented to symptoms, dysfunction, tension patterns, and osteopathic lesions, he began to recognize these as effects of deeper forces organizing them. He also learned to do less, or as poet Mary Oliver writes, "learning to be astonished." Craniosacral Biodynamics espouses this theme. In that every treatment session is unique, I find myself continually astonished, even while listening to and honoring how the client's potency guides the unfolding treatment program. This chapter explores some common ways for the treatment plan to present.

Sutherland's student Rollin Becker continued the investigation into the workings of potency Sutherland espoused. At one point, Becker realized that all his good osteopathic work was effective for some patients and not for others. He determined to just listen and do nothing until he understood what was actually happening, and learn from this how to be consistently effective as practitioner. After many sessions of just observing potency at work, he felt he understood. He perceived the healing process of potency, the inherent treatment program (or plan). In the words of Becker, "When you're dealing with the body's inherent forces, you've got to write a whole new set of rules for the game."[103] His focus was on supporting connection to the ever-present health in the client's system: "The purpose of the kind of care I give is strictly to allow your system to have all the resources that are available for it to work with … In other words, I'm treating to restore health; I'm not treating to correct the problem. In treating this way, I have opened the doors for the body to try to do what it wants to do with its own living forces."[104]

Craniosacral Biodynamics follows in the footsteps of these courageous and observant pioneers of Cranial Osteopathy. Rather than trying to figure out what is wrong and applying various techniques to try to fix it, we settle ourselves deeper in the dynamic stillness, honoring and resonating with the work and intelligence of the Breath of Life acting through potency. Sills writes:

> The inherent treatment plan orients us to the knowledge that the arising and sequencing of what has to happen in any given healing process is a function of primary respiration, not of practitioner analysis, and will unfold in its own way. Practitioners do not have to analyze or diagnose to learn what needs to happen, nor do they have to decide what to do, or how to intervene. They do, however, have to develop an inner state of stillness, orientation, and listening that opens a perceptual doorway to this intrinsic process.[105]

More biomechanical forms of healing approaches, including some other styles of Craniosacral Therapy, involve analyzing and assessing the location and nature of problems, and then applying various techniques to correct them. In Craniosacral Biodynamics, we are guided by our perception of holding patterns in the body, not to try to fix them but to orient to the forces organizing them. This leads us to sensing organizing points of stillness, or fulcrums, where unresolved conditional forces are contained (or "centered" as Becker called it) by potency.[106] A fulcrum is defined as a point of stillness around which movement organizes, as is discussed in detail in the following pages. Rather than taking it upon ourselves as practitioners to decide which fulcrum to work with, we listen for the Intelligence with a capital I to choose. This is the potency of the Breath of Life at work through the inherent treatment plan.

Where Sutherland's earlier work, based on his osteopathic training, involved active evaluative methods, like motion testing, to assess where motion was restricted or preferred, his later work was about deepening, quieting, and witnessing the potency do the work. We continue, informed by this legacy, as well as the additional clarifications of natural healing processes from Becker. Sills has further elucidated the inherent treatment plan and the functions of potency, rendering them more comprehensible and accessible to students and new practitioners. This chapter takes us on a tour of the inherent treatment plan in action.

A Paradigm Shift

Craniosacral Biodynamics can challenge our usual way of being and perceiving. Buddhist teacher Thich Nhat Hanh writes beautifully of the paradigm shift required of us for happiness. His words also apply to Craniosacral Biodynamics and our ability to perceive the unfolding of the inherent treatment plan:

> We often ask, "What's wrong?" Doing so, we invite painful seeds of sorrow to come up and manifest. We feel suffering, anger, and depression, and produce more such seeds. We would be much happier if we tried to stay in touch with the healthy, joyful seeds inside of us and around us. We should learn to ask, "What's not wrong?" and be in touch with that. There are so many elements in the world and within our bodies, feelings, perceptions, and consciousness that are wholesome, refreshing, and healing. If we block ourselves, if we stay in the prison of our sorrow, we will not be in touch with these healing elements.[107]

Students of our two-year foundation training in Craniosacral Biodynamics inevitably experience a paradigm shift at some point. The shift involves several aspects of how we perceive and practice in Craniosacral Biodynamics compared to the cultural norm in our modern Western world. One aspect of the shift is in widening and deepening our perception to sense wholeness and health. We practice immersing ourselves in tides and stillness in the ocean, rather than actively bouncing on the waves on the surface.

Where culturally we learn to focus in on an issue, to evaluate it, to analyze its exact expression, symptoms, language, etc., in Craniosacral Biodynamics, we learn to widen our perception to include as much of the whole as possible. We intend to view the issue as suspended within the whole. We practice perceiving the physical body not isolated in a void but as suspended within the fluid body, suspended within the larger field of radiance of the tidal body of long tide. And all of this is suspended within a potent field of dynamic stillness. The client is not there dangling within these fields alone. We are suspended together. Our boundaries as individuals become less important as we deepen and widen in our perception. From this perspective, we have fields within fields, an entire cosmos if you will, as resource. Returning to wholeness and source (resource), we have less need to solve the problem as individuals. Interestingly, in some languages (e.g., German) the words for *health* and *wholeness* are closely related. The word *heal* originally meant "to make whole."[108]

This is in stark contrast to the modern Western worldview, where separateness and individuality are encouraged, and where physicians and other health professionals are trained to assess problems and do what they can to fix them. I have heard that in traditional Chinese medicine, doctors would be paid only for keeping their patients well. If a patient became ill, the doctor had failed and would not be paid! This paradigm is more relevant to the osteopathic approach, originally laid out by A. T. Still, who wrote, "To find health should be the object of the physician. Anyone can find disease."[109]

If our job is to find health, we must let go of our need to fix what we believe is broken. It may represent health rather than deficiency. Becker points out that health is always present and active in the person's system:

> The seeking of health from within is a continuous time, tissue, and tidal effort from conception to the final moments of physiological life. Within every trauma and/or disease entity, there is an effort on the part of body physiology to deliver health mechanisms through the local area of stress to full functioning health capacities.[110]

We are always seeking health. We are always expressing it.

This implies that what we may perceive as problems, and what the client may complain about, are actually expressions of health, or at least the seeking of health. The paradigm shift includes being able to trust this. We tend to believe that health problems indicate a lack of health. Health has somehow gone into hiding or been used up. Can we trust that it is still present, even when we have trouble perceiving it? The long tide is always there, even when its expression is difficult to perceive due to the conditions of life. When Primary Respiration presents, it often feels to me like the sun coming out from behind the clouds. The sun is always there, even if the clouds prevent us from seeing it or feeling its warmth. It is also there at night, even if the earth itself is occluding its view. Can we trust that health is also omnipresent, always available, steadfastly with us? This is an underlying concept in working with the inherent treatment plan. Both of these important osteopathic principles, wholeness and the primacy of health, are essential background for understanding and supporting the unfolding of the inherent treatment plan.

This plan is by definition an expression of the Intelligence of the system in action. Intelligence with a capital I is a manifestation of health! Potency expresses health. It knows how to work with the conditions, traumas, and other external forces presented to it. It may have already worked for years to contain these forces, waiting for a time when the client's system has adequate resources available to complete processing and resolving them. Such a time can arise when the client rests in the safe relational field we as practitioners provide. Our ability to settle ourselves and support the client in settling can enable the client's system to deepen under the defensive activation clients so often arrive with. With this settling, the potency is free to do its healing work. Before we look more specifically at how the inherent treatment plan may unfold, let's first examine the three functions of potency, all essential to maintaining health and all apparent in the plan's unfolding.

Three Functions of Potency: Organizing, Protecting, and Healing

At the essence of Craniosacral Biodynamics is our perception, appreciation, and respect for forces underlying apparent form in health and disease. Becker identified potency as an inherent force acting within us, supporting our ability to meet conditions and the process of healing in relation to them:

> The body has the capacity to express health through this inherent potency. At the very core of total health there is a potency with the human body manifesting it in health. At the very core of every trauma or disease condition within the human body there is a potency manifesting its relationship with the body in trauma or disease. It is up to us to learn to feel this potency. It is relatively easy to feel the tensions and stresses of trauma and disease as they are manifesting their patterns. But within these manifesting elements there is a potency that is able "to control or influence, having authority or power." It centers the disturbance. It can be sensed and read by a feeling touch.[111]

In understanding the unfolding of the inherent treatment plan, it is helpful to become more acquainted with its director, potency. As Becker described potency, it has three functions, clarified by Sills as organizing, protecting, and healing.[112] All are relevant to the inherent treatment plan. The first is an organizing function. As noted earlier, our formation is guided by the Intelligence of potency. This is true both for the embryo forming in the womb and also throughout our lives. I have heard that our cells completely change every seven years. The exact period of seven years is questionable, as different kinds of cells live for different lengths of time. It is true, however, that our cells die and are replaced by other cells. Cells that originally formed my body as an embryo are no longer part of this body today, and the community of cells now making up my body has members who were not part of the community when I was born! Yet, my body persists with some degree of continuity. How does it know how to do this? How does my finger know how to heal each time I cut it while cooking?

What seems even more miraculous is that each of us turns out to have some kind of human form, each with our unique variations but all recognizable as human. In the midst of writing this chapter, I came across a moving, inspirational TED talk by Lizzie Velasquez, a young woman diagnosed as a baby with a very rare condition that prevented her from gaining any weight at all. She was expected to be dependent for life. Accused of being a monster by bullies in her teen years, her humanity persisted. She determined to become a motivational speaker, and also set other goals she has accomplished, achieving more than many at her young age of twenty-five (at the time of the talk).[113] She looks unusual but she is very human, despite the bullying and assumptions when she was younger. This is a brilliant demonstration of the miracle of life. Her life force shines through, even in the face of extreme physical differentness.

We all begin as one fertilized cell, a union of sperm and egg. Somehow, from this one cell, our remarkably functional bodies emerge and continue to emerge throughout our lives. Even those of us with malformations of different types (e.g., I have an extra rib; some people are missing an arm or leg, etc.) continue to form and re-form ourselves with some degree of continuity and function, enabling survival. How do we know how to do this? A mysterious force guides this process. This force is potency, transmuted from the Breath of Life.

Potency is a major biodynamic universal force organizing us as organisms. In Craniosacral Biodynamics we refer to an original blueprint guiding our development as a quantum field. If we met no adverse conditions in life, we would form entirely according to this blueprint. Regardless of what traumas or challenges we encounter, the blueprint remains, available to guide our cells and tissues in their organization via the work of potency. The conditions of life, however, also have their effects. Depending on how healthy and resourced we are at the time we meet them, conditional events may or may not be resolved as they occur. Conditional forces enter our field, applying their own organizational effects, often quite different from those of the original program. We do our best to adjust and accommodate. Potency in this case acts to protect us, its second important function. If a conditional force is too great to resolve at the time, potency spirals in around it to contain it. The tissues in the area tend to become denser and usually demonstrate reduced motility. Potency is holding them in a pattern, organized by a point of stillness. We call this organizing point of stillness an inertial fulcrum. In this case, the stillness relates to held conditional forces, reducing that fulcrum's ability to move and fully express Primary Respiration.

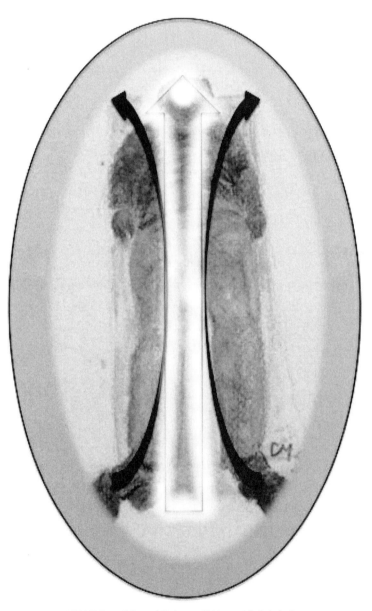

FIGURE 25: Natural Fulcrum Rising with Inhalation

Fulcrums are points of stillness organizing motion. The body organizes in relation to both inertial and natural fulcrums. The latter relate to the original blueprint or matrix. This matrix has a midline with points of stillness along it. When unaffected by conditional forces, the body naturally organizes in relation to these natural fulcrums. We also consider these to be automatically shifting fulcrums, as they move with each inhalation and exhalation of Primary Respiration. With the surging up the midline of inhalation at the mid-tide level, the natural fulcrums shift upward. With exhalation, they settle back down toward the tail or feet. The entire tissue-fluid-potency field moves with them as a holistic breathing of Primary Respiration.

Inertial fulcrums, on the other hand, do not move as easily with Primary Respiration and are often away from the midline. They are inertial, tending to stay put and resist motion. They can be sensed as points of relatively immobile density (an inertial stillness) within the unified fluid tissue field. There may be a sense of a pull toward or tension in relation to inertial fulcrums. While tissues organize in relation to natural fulcrums when not affected by trauma or other unresolved history, the presence of inertial fulcrums and conditional forces becomes an additional organizing influence. In their presence, we sense deviations from the midline-oriented filling and emptying of inhalation and exhalation. Usually, there is a pattern within the tissues, often experienced with some discomfort, pain, or dysfunction by the client. Clients tend to arrive with their attention on these problem areas. Our interest, however, is not on the pattern itself, which is an effect of the potency and conditional forces organizing it. We orient to the actual organizing center, with its organizing potency.

Becker wrote:

> My attention as a physician using diagnostic touch, is on the potency within this patient because I know if a change takes place within this potency, a whole new pattern will manifest itself, towards health for the patient. I know that there is a basic potency that can be found in the patient when he is in a state of health, and I know that when various energies that are present in traumatic or disease conditions have dissipated, there is a potency and a general feeling of biodynamic intrinsic forces manifesting themselves that tell me this patient is well again.[114]

Informed by a modern Western way of doing and acting, our tendency as practitioners is to look for the problem and how to fix it. Orienting to the underlying organizing forces involves shifting paradigms and perception. We then encounter a more inclusive view of health and wholeness. With this awareness, we can support the potency in its healing work. In this vein, we listen for *changes in the potency,* rather than focusing on the tissues and motion patterns. These are effects of the underlying potency and conditional forces the potency contains. It is the shifts in potency that inform us as to how the inherent treatment plan is unfolding.

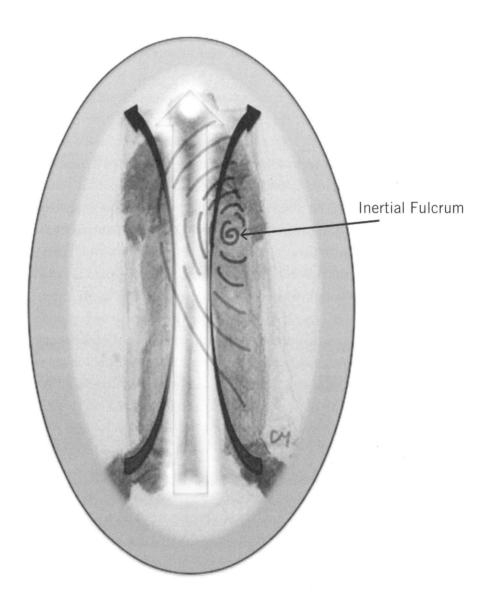

Inertial Fulcrum

FIGURE 26: Inertial Fulcrum Added to the System

Inertial Fulcrums: Health in Action

At the heart of an inertial site is potency that has the power to hold the added forces in check and organize them in the best possible way in the body physiology. This potency is a manifestation of the most basic ordering forces in the human system.[115]

Inertial fulcrums are areas where potency has coalesced to protect. The forces being contained by this protective coalescing and commonly accompanying tissue densification can result from any experience that has been too much or too intense for the system to integrate at the time. These include not only physical knocks, blows, or traumas, but also emotional or relational insults, traumas, and shocks, and even toxicity and genetic predispositions. Such influences can begin with birth or even as early as conception. The context within which we form affects our formation and serves as an organizational influence. If we are conceived through love, tenderness, and affection, our body-mind has different forces affecting it than if we are conceived through violence, rape, or alcoholic stupor.

I suspect one influence that enabled Lizzie Velasquez to succeed in her life and prove her doctors wrong about being able to be independent was the context her parents provided for her to grow in. Despite the doctor's warnings of how difficult life would be for Lizzie, they insisted on taking her home, loving her, and treating her as normal, to the extent that Lizzie had no idea until she started school at age five that she looked different from other children. The context of love and acceptance she developed in during her earliest years was an important organizational influence, helping to counterbalance the effect of whatever caused her unusual syndrome, as well as the cruelty of bullies she encountered in her teens. Similarly, when we hold our clients within an orientation to health and potency, we create a context where their health and potency are supported in shining through the clouds.

Potency is not just about physical issues. Our bodies and minds are intimately connected. Emotional and relational experiences are important forces in our lives and body-minds. Just as potency is less available when holding inertial fulcrums throughout the physical body, so we have less or altered relational energy available for maintaining or starting interpersonal or romantic relationships when we have unfinished business from previous relationships. These can be previous romantic relationships that have ended, earlier friendships, or familial or other relationships that had over-whelmingly challenging or traumatic aspects. Although psychotherapy is specific for working through relational issues like these, the work we do in Craniosacral Biodynamics in settling the relational field is crucial for enabling the client's system to work with its inertial fulcrums. This involves the healing function of potency essential to the inherent treatment plan. As we shall see, when the relational field has settled within a biodynamic session, the ground is set for the client's system to deepen under all its history, patterns, and activations. In this supportive context, the potency can then begin to interact with unresolved conditional forces so they can be resolved and released, revealing the health and wholeness that has been waiting to shine.

No matter what we have experienced, if we are alive, health and wholeness persist. Mindfulness teacher Jon Kabat-Zinn speaks to this eloquently, although he does not use the term *potency:*

> Wholeness and connectedness are what are most fundamental in our nature as living beings. No matter how many scars we carry about from what we have gone through and suffered in the past, our intrinsic wholeness is still here: what else contains the scars? None of us has to be a helpless victim of what was done to us or what was not done for us in the past, nor do we have to be helpless in the face of what we may be suffering now. We are also what was present before the scarring, our original wholeness, what was born whole. And we can reconnect up with our intrinsic wholeness at any time because its very nature is that it is always present.[116]

In meeting inertial fulcrums, it is important to understand that they contain not only conditional forces left over from an unresolved experience; they also hold potency, the biodynamic, universal force of life, which is acting there in its protective mode to contain the conditional forces. Take a moment to remember the slime mold discussed in the previous chapter. When the researcher, Seifritz, injects a toxin into the protoplasm, its flow stops in the local area, but continues elsewhere. Seifritz concludes, "Thus the protoplasm meets contingencies, heals itself, and thus saves itself." When faced with anesthesia, the protoplasm suddenly stops flowing, which Seifritz points out, "could occur only if the protoplasm has solidified."[117] This is an example of the coalescing of potency at an inertial fulcrum affecting the fluid and tissue it organizes. Note that the potency coalesces first; the tissues solidify in response.

If we perceive a pattern or area of density or inertia, our intention is not to change or fix the problem. Rather, in Craniosacral Biodynamics, we orient to the organizing forces affecting the area perceived. These include both universal biodynamic forces of potency and the conditional forces the potency is containing. Understanding the pattern to be an effect of the actions of these underlying forces, we listen for a sense of what is organizing or generating the pattern or tissue compression we perceive. Where is the point of stillness serving as its organizing fulcrum, the inertial fulcrum? For example, in figure 27, we see a common inertial pattern in the cranium, referred to as side-bending. Orienting to the forces from which this altered sense of motion in the cranial base results, we become aware of an inertial fulcrum within the spheno-basilar junction, the joint between the sphenoid and the basilar part of the occiput.

Referring to osteopathic lesions, the classical osteopathic term for holding areas or patterns in the tissues, Becker writes, "Osteopathic lesions are effects that are found in body physiology. When you find an osteopathic lesion, you must consider in your thinking these primary factors. Consider the energy field that was poured into the patient from without, and also consider the factors from within the patient, in their

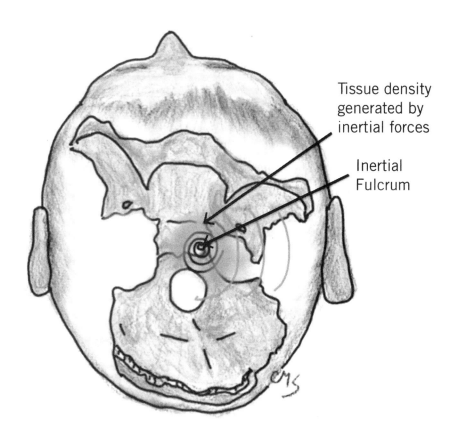

Tissue density generated by inertial forces

Inertial Fulcrum

FIGURE 27: Inertial Fulcrum Organizing Tissue Pattern

own conscious thinking and nervous system, that are leading their body to create this energy field. You've got to combine all of it."[118]

In this vein, we understand that the inertial pattern and its fulcrum are an expression of health and Intelligence. If we decide to apply some technique to change it, the tissues may shift. The forces within the fulcrum, however, generally remain unresolved and are likely to express elsewhere as another problem or pain. Furthermore, if we just address the pattern we perceive, we may be upsetting a larger compensatory design we are ignorant of, adding additional forces with our good intentions. I have heard of a case where a well-meaning practitioner worked on changing a tension pattern, resulting in the symptom disappearing. The next day, however, the client committed suicide! The pattern that had been holding the person together enabling him to manage in life was suddenly gone. He could not cope without it. Listening to the inherent treatment plan, regardless of what we think should or shouldn't happen or be addressed next, enables the Intelligence to address issues within the context of the whole. All aspects of the system can adjust to the changes as potency supports them in ways we as individuals outside the system might not be able to. As an embodied expression of long tide within the fluid-tissue field, potency is in touch with the whole of the individual and can work on many levels at once, while we might not even be aware of them!

Doing our best to leave our little ego needs behind, resting in the support of source, we trust the tide to its work. Our aim as practitioners is to orient to the organizing forces and so support the potency in completing its protective function and being able to apply its healing function through the unfolding of the inherent treatment plan.

The Inherent Treatment Plan Unfolds

The inherent treatment plan can unfold in different ways, expressing within long tide, mid-tide, or dynamic stillness, or some combination thereof, but we know it is unlikely to clarify if the client does not feel safe and settled within the relational field. This is a major reason the relational field and its settling is so emphasized in this approach. Sills has delineated the stages of the inherent treatment plan as follows, as a way to support practitioners perceiving and facilitating it through their aware presence.

A diagram of the inherent treatment plan unfolding is shown on the following page.[119]

In exploring the inherent treatment plan, we understand that deep healing work does not occur at the level of the CRI. Work at this level tends to be more locally focused. Without accessing the resources of the larger fields we are suspended within

THE INHERENT TREATMENT PLAN

The First Settling

The Relational Field

The practitioner orients to Primary Respiration and the relational field is negotiated and settles.

The Second Settling:

The Holistic Shift

As the practitioner settles into a receptive state oriented to Primary Respiration and to the client's midline and three bodies, a shift from conditions and the CRI level of expressions occurs and deepens. It is from this holistic shift that healing intentions meditated by the Breath of Life emerge.

Holistic shift deepens and the Long Tide clarifies as healing intentions emerge as an expression of Long Tide phenomenon.	←→ Holistic shift deepens and healing intentions emerge within the fluid and physical bodies mediated by the tidal potencies. Becker's three phases of (1) seeking, (2) settling into a state of balance/dynamic equilibrium,	←→ Holistic shift deepens into dynamic stillness and healing intentions emerge within and from a ground of emergence that is both dynamic and vibrantly alive.

(3) reorganization and realignment.

© Franklyn Sills 2016

and the Intelligence of potency, work at this faster CRI level can be overwhelming and even traumatizing. Although symptoms may change, the deeper forces creating them are often not addressed at the CRI level. They remain in the system, causing old symptoms to reappear or new ones to arise. Furthermore, because the CRI is associated with conditions of life, addressing issues on this surface level of the ocean can easily stir up the frequently intense emotions and sensations of past traumas and experiences. We find that the potency is generally unable to perform its deeper healing work until the client's system has settled under all of these activations related to trauma and conditions. We observe activity on the CRI level, and continue to deepen and widen our perception to include more of the whole, where we can more easily access resource and potency with which to resolve the forces underlying the issue in a more gentle and inclusive manner. We begin by settling with the client as two human beings meeting within our relational field.

Settling of the Relational Field

Until basic trust is established, nothing of any depth can occur.[120]

The inherent treatment plan begins with the settling of the relational field, as the plan is unlikely to unfold without this, with potency remaining in its protective function. As discussed in chapter 3, the relationship between practitioner and client is an important context within which healing can occur. Clients arrive with their relational history in tow and may readily transfer old relational issues onto the relationship with the practitioner. It is important for practitioners to be present in a state of being, supporting being-to-being interaction, rather than meeting the client from a reactive egotistic self state. From this state of being, there is more direct access to source. The Breath of Life can more easily be sensed. As we as practitioners settle and resource ourselves, we are more able to support this process in the client, facilitating a sense of trust and safety.

One aspect of settling the relational field involves our physical contact. Our careful negotiation with the client to establish comfortable, relaxing touch supports the client in being able to trust us. It is not unusual for clients to have experienced touch that felt invasive, disrespectful, or even traumatic in the past. They may have had other bodyworkers or health practitioners making uncomfortable contact. In many medical procedures, for example, contact is not comfortable. It takes a special bedside manner that many practitioners don't demonstrate, particularly in stressful emergency medical situations, to enable the patient to have any sense of comfort or safety while being poked with a needle, prodded in an examination, or moved from one position to another. Clients may have experienced rough or insensitive handling when in a horizontal, dependent state, similar to their position on the treatment table. Unfortunately, being handled in an impersonal, insensitive way is a common aspect of birth trauma. While the client may not consciously remember such an early experience, the body may react to sudden shifts in contact or being touched in certain places or without warning as if the experience were happening again.

It is helpful to let the client know you are about to make or shift contact, to check in as to how the contact feels, and to encourage clients to let you know if anything is uncomfortable. I explain to new clients that it is extremely important to me that they are comfortable with my touch and in general during the session because the work has so much to do with settling. It is difficult to settle if you don't feel comfortable or safe. I try to help the client be as comfortable and safe as possible. If the client doesn't feel safe, even if at a tissue level rather than consciously, the nervous system will activate defensively. The amygdala will warn the system of danger. The sympathetic nervous system will accelerate things in preparation for fight or flight. Simply talking softly and gently to the client may help with settling or deepening under after defensive reactions, as the social engagement system comes online and safety can be detected in present time within this current relational field.

Another important aspect of negotiation involves the energetic space between practitioner and client. With physical contact, we negotiate how firm or soft to make the contact, the exact positioning, etc. Our touch tends to be more comfortable if we stabilize our hands. We can use our elbows as fulcrums by making sure they are supported by the treatment table, cushions, etc. Then the stillness of those fulcrums is transmitted through our hands. These physical aspects of contact are important. There is also an energetic component, which clients are often less aware of. Biodynamic practitioners learn to sense and adjust their attentional distance, which we began exploring in chapter 3. A client's system may feel intruded upon if our attention is too close. It is not unusual for students and new practitioners to get "too interested" in a phenomenon they perceive or are learning to perceive. Their attention narrows in on the structure or fulcrum or whatever it is they are interested in. The client's fluid body may react by going still or hiding. This stillness is different from dynamic stillness. Protective stilling is more like freezing. It is inert, feeling dead, absent, or empty. There may also be activation in the system, sensed as motion patterns, pulsations, or fluctuations. These are reactions to the external force coming from the practitioner's attention. The client may feel discomfort with this kind of attention. Complaints of headaches or other aches or pains are not unusual, as well as feeling sped up, anxious, and unable to settle.

It is helpful for the practitioner to be able to back off in these situations. This usually means widening attention, grounding by sensing one's feet or sacrum, orienting to midline, and returning to a sense of being suspended within the three bodies with an orientation to wholeness and Primary Respiration. It may be useful to think of shifting your attention, as if you were viewing from behind yourself a few inches or feet, or even from a greater distance such as from down the road or in the next city. Usually, however, thinking of dropping down in your own body, or even a sense of roots reaching into the earth, and widening the attention are what is called for.

It is also possible for attention to be too distant. There is a sense of the client reaching out, looking for you. The client may even say, "I don't feel you. Where are you?" In this case, it is important to experiment with bringing your attention in a bit at a time, maintaining a wide field of perception but coming in closer until you and the client have a sense of meeting. This kind of negotiation is often life-changing for clients with relational or touch trauma histories. I have had clients tearfully expressing their appreciation for my careful negotiation, declaring, "No one has ever asked before!" Inquiring into the contact and attentional distance that feels right can be profoundly healing and settling. Like Goldilocks exploring the home of the three bears, it is a process of finding what feels "just right." Then we can settle within our relational field.

Unfortunately, Goldilocks, and the old woman who historically preceded her in the original fairy tale, was intrusive, rather than relationally respectful. Understandably, the three bears were upset when they returned home to find their porridge eaten, their chairs sat upon and one broken, and an intruder sleeping in one of their beds. Goldilocks woke up and ran away. No relationship! Our clients may have had experiences of intrusion that felt like this. Or they may have run away like the little girl. The relational field we establish with the client is different, but may stir old memories of earlier relational traumas. It is important to enter this relational territory with care and awareness, enabling something different, safer, and more trustworthy to develop.

The relational field takes varying amounts of time and attention to settle. Some people are ready to trust you the moment they meet you. I find many of my clients arrive the first time already having a good sense of who I am from reading my website. I make a point of expressing myself as honestly and personally as possible while still being professional, in support of establishing trust easily. Clients with a relational trauma history, however, may have a much more difficult time settling within our relational field. Even if the trauma wasn't relational, the defensive autonomic nervous system activations set off by overwhelming trauma and shock can become the person's modus operandi. The social engagement system may be sleeping, so to speak, needing additional prompting to come out and play, as we will discuss in chapter 7 on working with trauma. In that such trauma is so often associated with the kinds of physical issues clients come to us with, it is not unusual to encounter difficulty settling the relational field. In my own practice, where I work extensively with stress and trauma, attention to the relational field settling becomes essential and at times primary.

At some point, the relational field settles. It may take minutes or months, depending on the client's history, as well as how we as practitioners are able to meet them. This settling occurs in part as we are talking with the client in our initial history taking, welcoming, and arriving, before the client is even on the treatment table. Then I usually take some time guiding settling on the table and settling myself deeper in relationship to the client. There is often a sense here, even more than when we were initially talking, of the field between us settling and deepening. There begins to be more of a perception of nonseparation or connectedness between us. Our fields are interacting. There is a feeling of quieting as we deepen together. At this point, I negotiate making physical contact, where the settling can continue.

The Holistic Shift

Becker advised his students to do nothing until they sensed wholeness and Primary Respiration.[121] Sills termed this change from conditions to inherent wholeness and the deeper tidal expression the "holistic shift." In some forms of cranial work, this sense of deeper settling is the end point. After addressing all the presenting patterns, lesions, etc., the system might seem more settled. In our work, however, this is really the starting point. Our intention is to support the client's system in settling under the patterns and conditions, to reconnect with the deeper stillness and Breath of Life. We support this primarily through resonance and attention to resource. Deepening our own state as practitioners into Primary Respiration and dynamic stillness makes this more available to the client's system. It is as if our being in stillness communicates to the client's system and reminds it that stillness is the ground of being, always present and waiting. Research demonstrates that when two systems come into contact with each other, the more coherent one tends to influence the other toward more coherence.[122] This seems to be one way the practitioner facilitates settling in the client.

We also support the client's settling through the not-doing that accompanies our resting by being in stillness. Understanding that any intention on our part to change something in the client's system may be perceived by the client's fluid body as an external, possibly intrusive force to be managed, we do not attempt to change any-thing. We settle deeply within ourselves, orienting initially to our own midline and three-body suspensory system. When we have a sense of this settling within ourselves (which hopefully is established before the client arrives!), we then widen our attention to include the client. The client's midline then becomes the center of our field of per-ception. We intend to sense the client's physical body as suspended within the wider fluid body of the client suspended within the field of radiance of the long tide sus-pended within dynamic stillness. We notice whatever patterns may present as we con-tinue to orient to the wider, deeper fields and the action of potency within those fields.

Our initial contact with the client's physical body is usually at the feet as a place that most people find grounding, soothing, and safe. Often, with this first contact, we sense pulsations, pulls, tension, patterns, relatively chaotic motions, to-ing and fro-ing, and various rapid motions relating to CRI. These are compensatory pat-terns, ways the body has adapted to the challenges, conditions, and traumas it has encountered. Rather than engaging with these patterns or focusing on them, which can reinforce them or interfere with the inherent intentions of potency, we acknowl-edge their presence and continue to deepen, widen, and orient to the underlying stillness. We also check in with the client, supporting them as needed to orient to the resources, to settle into a sense of breath, to the support of the treatment table under them, the sensation of our contact, and other sensations. We aim to support the client in settling, calming, resting. With physical contact may arise new levels of relational field activation. We support communication as needed, staying in present time, orienting to safety.

As the client is able to orient to safety in present time, the more chaotic motions begin to settle. There may be waves of nervous system discharge, usually sensed as rapid pulsations or buzzing, followed by deeper settling. Things begin to feel softer, less tense, smoother, slower. As this settling occurs, there is often a sense of wholeness. Where we may initially be aware of just the feet, as in figure 28a, they begin to feel more connected up the legs to the trunk, the heart, eventually the whole body. Often the client also comments on this sense of connectedness.

With the wholeness there is often a sense of midline and supportive energetic fields clarifying, as in figure 28b. Then we may notice motion oriented to the midline. Often the mid-tide expresses at this point. There is a sense of widening out from midline, fol-lowed by a narrowing back in toward it as the whole fluid body fills and empties with

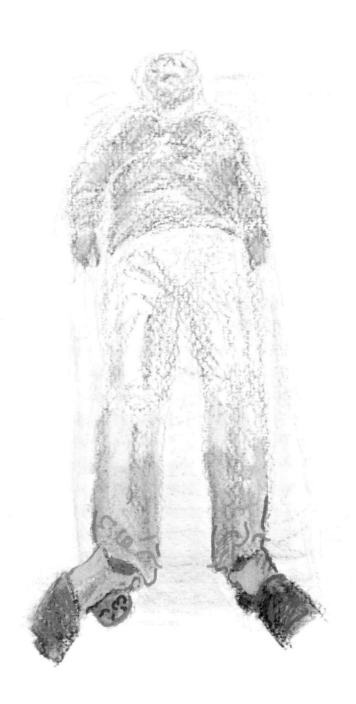

FIGURE 28A: Holistic Shift
Before the holistic shift has begun

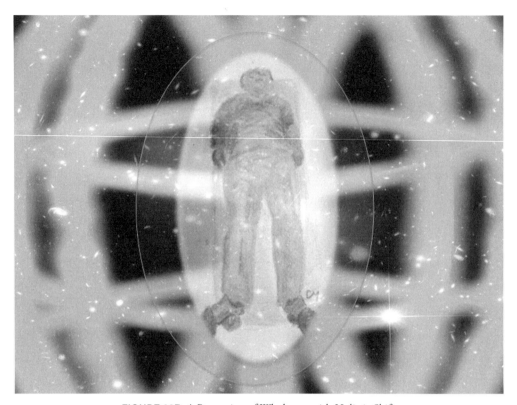

FIGURE 28B: A Perception of Wholeness with Holistic Shift

inhalation and exhalation of mid-tide. While this may be a subtle sense of mid-tide initially, with the CRI motions still apparent, with deeper settling the tide or Primary Respiration becomes clearer and stronger, as if coming out from behind the clouds. (Dynamic stillness rather than tidal motion may present.) The CRI motions become less apparent. Again, there may be waves of nervous system discharge and deeper levels of settling.

This sense of wholeness and Primary Respiration arising represents the holistic shift. It is not a precise moment in time but rather a process occurring over some period. It may take ten minutes or it may take several sessions to arrive at, depending on how settled the relational field is between practitioner and client, how resourced the client is, and how much experience both client and practitioner have had with Cranio-sacral Biodynamics. It can take practice for the client's system to orient to something other than pattern. Remember, this is a paradigm shift. Clients often arrive very fixated on their problems. Their mindset can have a strong effect on their ability to settle and access the Intelligence within.

Once the holistic shift has arisen, however long it takes, we then begin to perceive the inherent treatment plan unfolding more specifically. The potency is then not pre-occupied with defensive stances. It no longer needs to protect against the practitioner's input as an intrusive external force. It need not remain caught up with reacting to all of its history. There is an ability to communicate more directly with source, with the Breath of Life. In this more settled, holistic state, we sense the potency making decisions about what to work with next. We may perceive many patterns with their many inertial fulcrums organizing them as one interconnected network, all part of a holistic compensatory system managed by potency. A sense of intention then arises, as if the potency is focusing on one particular inertial fulcrum and for the moment letting go of all the others. One particular inertial fulcrum becomes uncoupled from its connection with rest. The potency of the entire system is now available to work with this one fulcrum.

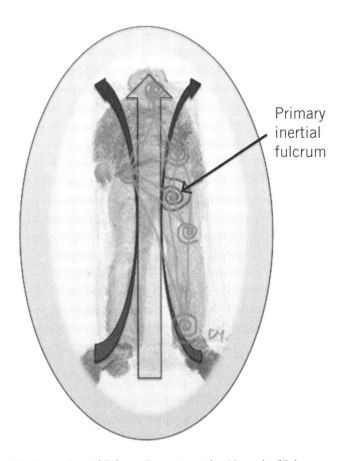

Primary inertial fulcrum

FIGURE 29: Inertial Fulcrum Presenting within Network of Fulcrums

As practitioners, we may feel at this stage pulled or drawn to a certain area. This is quite different from the desire we may have before holistic shift occurs to move to work with different tension patterns presenting in the client. Prior to the holistic shift, the potency has not yet made a choice of where to work. Its healing intention has not yet emerged. If we as practitioners make the choice at that stage, we are likely acting from an egotistic need to do something, to fix the problem, to be perceived as a perceptive, knowledgeable practitioner, etc. Sills writes, "This intention arises as a function of the inherent forces present and is not a function of practitioner analysis or intervention. It cannot be figured out or motion tested for and, indeed, any intervention by the practitioner at this point will undercut the whole process."[123]

Being with the unknown in this way may stimulate insecurity within us. It takes trust, patience, and deepening to wait and listen for a sense of wholeness and Primary Respiration coming to the fore. Once holistic shift has arrived, we may sense a particular fulcrum lighting up. It may seem as if the fluid-tissue field distorts around a particular area, with the tissue motility with each phase of primary inhalation and exhalation being limited or altered in this area. Potency, as an embodied life force within the fluids, may seem to shift toward a fulcrum or permeate the given area. At the long-tide level, there may be a sense of a windlike motion as potency shifts toward the fulcrum in question. The fulcrum and its pattern clarify, as if coming forward in a crowd or emerging from the background of a fulcrum-composed web. We can perceive the fulcrum as being suspended within the fields within fields of the whole three-body suspensory system. Sills writes, "Now all fields of action—potency, fluids, and tissues—are oriented to a particular fulcrum, issue, and healing potential. As this occurs, all other inertial fulcrums recede into the background and the fulcrum being attended to can be safely dealt with without overwhelming the system or the person involved."[124]

We are sensing the potency choosing that particular fulcrum to work with. It is not about my personal choice as practitioner. It is important for us as practitioners to essentially get out of the way, to listen deeply, if we intend to support the potency in its work. Once potency has chosen a fulcrum to work with, we may feel drawn to move our hands to be in more direct contact with that particular fulcrum. As the potency has already oriented to this fulcrum, our listening presence can serve as supportive augmentation of what is already happening.

The Breath of Life is free to act according to its Intelligence without our interference as the inherent treatment plan unfolds. Its healing intention may be apparent at the level of potency, fluids, and tissues arising from any level. It is common for it to arise as a mid-tide phenomenon, engaging embodied forces, directed by potency. We will continue our exploration here at the mid-tide level of perception, although it may also arise from within a long-tide level or dynamic stillness, or may shift from one level to another. This makes sense when we remember that potency is transmutation of the Breath of Life at the embodied level of mid-tide. It is not separate from any other expressions of the Breath of Life.

The Inherent Treatment Plan in Mid-Tide: Becker's Three-Step Process

Becker described three steps, or stages of awareness, common in the inherent treatment plan unfolding as healing intentions emerge at the mid-tide level. Sills has named these three steps seeking, settling and stilling, and reorganization and realignment.[125, 126]

Seeking

As described previously, we can sense the potency selecting a fulcrum to work with in various ways. As the fulcrum is chosen, the forces within it, both potency and conditional forces, are seeking dynamic equilibrium or a state of balance. We may sense fluid fluctuations or rocking around the area. If we focus in on the fluctuating motions or its related tissue pattern, we can augment the seeking activities and actually interfere with the underlying forces settling into a state of balance. Settling ourselves as practitioners further, widening our perception to hold the fulcrum within the whole field, or fields suspended within fields, we support the forces in also stilling. The potency at this stage is able to begin shifting from protective to healing function.

Settling and Stilling

As the forces within the inertial fulcrum settle into a state of balance, we enter the second phase Becker identified. Here, we sense stillness in all three bodies, in potency, fluids, and tissues, as the forces have settled. Becker described this state as follows: "A still pause-rest period, the potency, is reached, at which time all motion apparently ceases … When the pattern goes *through* the stillness, a change takes place within the potency. 'Something happens' as a result of this change in potency. This is the corrective phase of the treatment program."[127]

During this phase, our task as practitioners is to orient to the stillness and observe the "something" happening. As this occurs, potency shifts from a protective coalescence to a more vibrant healing process. We may sense energy being released, pulsations, heat, nervous system clearing, traumatic force vectors, or other sensations emitting from the fulcrum as the conditional forces that have been centered there are discharged, dissipating and returning to the field. Students of Craniosacral Biodynamics learn various methods to support this process if the state of balance isn't able to deepen. Once it has and there is a sense of resolution of the forces held within the fulcrum, something else happens. We then begin to sense the entire system reorganizing and realigning now that it doesn't have to organize in relation to this particular fulcrum.

Reorganization and Realignment

This is the third step of the three-step process, where the potency shifts into its organizational function. Various motions may be sensed as the entire three-body suspensory system rearranges itself in relation to the natural fulcrums along the midline, where previously it had to organize in relation to the inertial fulcrum. With this fulcrum dissolved, and the potency that was centering it liberated, we often sense a stronger drive or strength in the mid-tide, as well as more ease of motility with the tide in the area affected by the fulcrum. The cells and tissues can breathe more readily with the tidal inhalation and exhalation once the inertial fulcrum restricting them has resolved. As the system reorganizes, there is often a sense of mid-tide resuming, although at any point during this three-step process, the system may deepen into long tide or dynamic stillness and continue its work from there.

The Inherent Treatment Plan in Long Tide and Dynamic Stillness

Where the mid-tide is an embodied expression of the Breath of Life with potency acting as a powerful organizing, protective, and healing force within the fluids, long tide has a more airy and fiery quality. It is in a sense more about space and energy than about embodied form, although potency is also about energy, or "bioenergy," as Becker called it.[128]

At the level of long tide, an inertial fulcrum being chosen feels different than at the mid-tide level. There may be a sense of windlike forces or radiant light entering the system from some mysterious place outside the body. They may seem to enter the midline, work on a specific fulcrum, usually with quick resolution, and then move on to another fulcrum or to return to the vast field from whence it came. It is powerful, purposeful, and Intelligent. Again, the practitioner's role is to deepen, resonate, and witness in a supportive way. There is not much to do here! Often at a long-tide level, the client also feels deeply settled. Remember that long tide is not affected by personal history. Working at this level, the client is unlikely to be overwhelmed by past trauma.

There is usually more of a sense of peace and coherence. As fulcrums are resolved, the entire system reorganizes and realigns, as with mid-tide healing processes. From long tide, there may also be a sense of potency arising to work within the more embodied level of mid-tide and fluid body. This is not a linear, delineated process. The three bodies or fields are intertwined, one suspended within the other, each being a stepping down or transmutation of another. The treatment plan can easily move between these levels. As practitioners, it is helpful to be able to hold and witness the process by resting in dynamic stillness, being able to perceive and meet each level as it presents.

At any point, the system may deepen into dynamic stillness. The inherent treatment plan can unfold from within dynamic stillness as it interacts with embodied form, including inertial fulcrums. The healing process here does not lend itself easily to verbal description, as it is even less linear and form-oriented than at the mid-tide and long-tide levels. There is a sense of something happening or having happened in the stillness. Upon emerging from the stillness, it becomes apparent that various inertial fulcrums have resolved, although the exact steps of their resolution may not be obvious.

Dynamic stillness can have a sense of emptiness, even darkness, or profound lightness, where details of form are no longer apparent or important. It is as if they come back into form in a different way upon emerging from the stillness. My sense is that in stillness our form dissolves and can then re-form differently.

Dynamic stillness may come forward and recede during the session. Issues may be resolved during the stillness. Mid-tide with its potency or long tide with its windlike or light forces may then arise and continue with the healing process. Often, there is a return to mid-tide as the Intelligence completes its treatment plan for this time, and the system returns to a more embodied state, ready to engage with the outside world again. The return of the tide is often an indication that a process has completed. The strength, or drive, of the tide, as well as how symmetrical its expression is, demonstrates how the healing intentions of the inherent treatment plan have shifted motility within the client.

Meditation on the Inherent Treatment Plan

A guided exploration within your own body can give you a sense of how the treatment plan might unfold. You may want to record this exploration in your own voice and play it back to yourself to help you settle more deeply. (A recording is available at www.birthingyourlife.org/the-breath-of-life-book.)

Allow yourself to settle in a comfortable position, as in our previous explorations. Take note as you settle of the sensations informing you. What tells you that you are comfortable or not? Which parts of your body are you aware of or not? Are there areas of discomfort? Are there areas that feel good or OK? What is your breath like as you settle? What speaks to you of settling as you sit quietly?

You may find yourself becoming quieter, perhaps with a sense of softening, melting into the surface you are sitting on, breathing slowing and deepening. What supports you in being able to settle and feel safe in this moment? What is a resource for you in this process? What helps you to settle more fully just now?

As you continue to settle, let yourself become curious about your sense of wholeness. How much of the whole of you can you be aware of in this moment? Does your body present to you as parts, as a hand, a knee, a shoulder? Or do you begin to have a sense of these parts being connected? If so, where in your body is the sense of connection? Can you sense within the whole of your body a center-line running vertically from the base of your spine up through your head? We call this midline. What speaks to you of midline just now? This may be a physical sense of your spine, the boney midline. It may be a fluidic sense of flow. It may be a sense of light shining up and down the center of your body. What do you sense when you inquire into midline?

Allowing yourself to rest in this sense of wholeness and midline, let yourself be curious about any sense of motion or stillness within your body. If there is an area of discomfort, can you allow it to be part of the whole without focusing in on it? Let your awareness widen out from midline to the edges of your physical body, and, if you are comfortable without losing a sense of grounded presence, out beyond the physical. You may have a sense of an oval-shaped field around you. You may even feel like you are floating or suspended within this fluid field, like a little embryo supported within its amniotic sac. If this is a troubling image for you, let it go, but use it if it is helpful in feeling more settled and fluid. You may notice a sense of widening and narrowing in a slow rhythm, about twelve to fifteen cycles per minute. This fluid tide often includes a sense of building, surging up the midline, filling of the whole fluid body in inhalation, followed by a settling down and in toward midline, a receding, emptying sensation in exhalation. Don't worry if you don't sense anything like this. It takes practice to sense it, and the fluid tide may be in stillness.

If you are able to rest in this wider state of wholeness, let yourself become curious about what else you sense in your body. What draws your attention? Again, if there is an area of discomfort, can you just observe it as part of the whole, without narrowing your attention in on it? Without trying to change it? Let yourself simply observe your experience and see what unfolds. Be cautious of any tendency to follow any movement or sensation you become aware of. Can you hold whatever it is in your wide field of awareness, suspended within the oval of your fluid body, with its organizing midline in the center?

Be patient with your experience. This is not about trying to accomplish or change anything. Your task is to practice settling, perceiving, and being with what you perceive.

Stay with this as long as it is of interest to you. When you feel you are complete with the experience, notice what tells you that. The changes you notice are likely to be an expression of an inherent treatment within your own system.

When you feel done, take some time to sense your physical body. Press your feet into the floor, take a few deep breaths, then gently open your eyes, look around the room to orient yourself.

Take some notes to help you remember and integrate your experience.

Please be careful not to judge or criticize your experience in any way. You may find your attention wandered, or that you fell asleep. This may have been exactly what you needed at the time! Can you be open to the possibility of something useful happening here? Being with the inherent treatment plan requires letting go of what we think we know and what we think should happen. It is a humbling and enriching experience.

6
Formative Forces
Accessing Original Embryological Potential

*T*he session has been unfolding with gentle clarity. After settling into holistic shift, a sense of wholeness and some mid-tide arising, potency beckons me to a fulcrum in the left hip area. My client has arrived with complaints about a headache, and I can sense a pattern involving her cranial base, with some compression on the left side. As I listen from the feet, I begin to feel the entire fluid body moving in relation to the left hip, as if someone has pinched the fabric of the field there, restricting the movement. This fulcrum at the hip comes clearly into focus, as if emerging from a background where all other patterns and fulcrums drop out of view. As the hip fulcrum clarifies, I have a sense of to-ing and fro-ing of the fluids around it.

Listening to the draw of the potency as it chooses the hip fulcrum, I move from the feet to hold the hip gently with one hand in front and one behind. Here the seeking of the forces within the fulcrum settle out of their rocking, pulsating motions, and there is a sense of stilling. I begin to feel heat pouring out into my hand at the back of the hip, then a softening and spreading. Another wave of heat comes with some pulsations. I note a sense of connection with the sympathetic chain up either side of the spine, as if this fulcrum relates to a fight-or-flight pattern. I sense the left side of the head and neck as coalesced within this arrangement. Evidently, the same inertial forces held in the hip fulcrum are affecting the head and neck region, and the sympathetic chain seems to be involved.

As the tissues under my hand melt, the pattern begins to seem less relevant. I sense that the inertial forces held in the fulcrum have now completed discharging, as the heat and pulsations have calmed and there is now more of a sense of ease and fluid space. I sense more space opening in the head and neck area and a softening of the sympathetic chain.

Then a very sweet moment arises. I begin to feel like I am holding a little embryo within its fluid sac in the womb. I become aware of a strong sense of pull up from my hands toward the head. I realize I am sensing the primal midline coming into view. This is the energetic midline along which the primitive streak and then the notochord form within the embryo. All the cells and tissues of the embryo organize in relation to this midline and now I am feeling this happening within my client. The midline lights up for me, as if stepping center stage into the limelight. I sense it spiraling, rising up through the bodies of the vertebrae, where remnants of the notochord are believed to remain in the centers of the vertebral discs. This uprising feels almost fiery as it rushes up the midline. Various less coherent motions I have been sensing around the body through this reorganization phase now seem to settle as the tissues remember they can relate to the primal midline. I have a sense of a tiny embryo in my hands, beginning to lengthen, sprouting little arms and legs, growing a heart, a face, a brain, and a nervous system, all within my holding. My heart softens and glows in resonance with this miracle of life, repeating itself once again in my treatment room.

How life begins is highly relevant to our work with Craniosacral Biodynamics, as well as to every moment of our existence. Craniosacral Biodynamics is based on a perceptual understanding that the same universal forces guiding our formation in the womb continue to affect us throughout our lives. Our health and well-being depend on how our cells and tissues form and re-form in relation to these forces. In biodynamic session work, we perceive the effects of other, conditional forces being resolved as the inherent treatment plan unfolds. In the process, there is often a sense of the client's system returning to an embryonic state. It may even seem like we are holding a tiny embryo coming into form. Understanding the embryological forces involved, we can facilitate the system in orienting to these early universal forces to support health. In this chapter, we explore how we form as a transmutation, or stepping down, from the Breath of Life, manifesting within a vast field of light, with a local torus-shaped bioelectric field and "primal midline." A torus is a donut-shaped field with a hollow axis, or midline, and within this coherent energetic field, energy flows in one end, through the axis, and out the other end. (See figure 30A.)

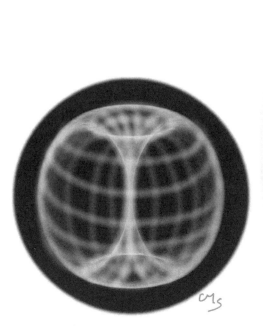

FIGURE 30A: Torus

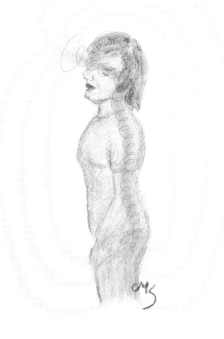

FIGURE 30B: Primal Midline within Torus

A Field of Light Ignites

Imagine, if you will, that at conception a field of light "ignites," drawing the slow, mysterious long tide toward the watery fertilized ovum, or "conceptus." As long tide is drawn in, a local torus-shaped bioelectric ordering field is generated within the larger tidal body of long tide. The torus spirals around a constantly uprising centerline we call the "primal midline." Within this energetic torus the conceptus is suspended and the miracle of embryological development unfolds.

Exciting new research may scientifically confirm this ignition of light as the sperm enters the ovum.[129] Scientists have found a way to see the moment an egg is "activated" at conception by using fluorescent indicators.[130] The brightness of the spark created through this process, which relates to physiological changes in the egg at the moment of conception, is apparently associated with the likelihood of survival of eggs observed during in vitro fertilization. Does this relate to the perception of ignition we experience in Craniosacral Biodynamics? We similarly sense the strength of the ignition, which we perceive at the end of each exhalation or beginning of inhalation of long tide, to be related to health.

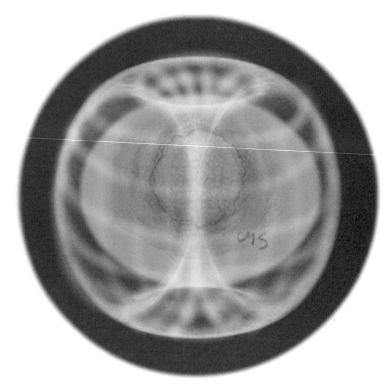

FIGURE 31: Early Embryo within Torus

In session work, we may experience a sense of a sudden lighting up of the field of long tide. It is as if a mysterious light energy is being transferred from the field into the fluids, where we can have a sense of a surge of potency in response to the ignition. As mentioned earlier, Sills has described a field of light being established at conception, as an original matrix is laid down.[131] Within this field, a local bioelectric ordering field is generated. We perceive this local field as a further stepping down from the Breath of Life. This torus-shaped bioelectric field is slightly more coalesced, closer to physical manifestation, than the field of light, which we also call the quantum field. While the field of light has a midline, which we call the "quantum midline," the torus has its own "primal midline," which is the path along which the first midline appears in the little embryo as the primitive streak fourteen days after conception. Let's get to know this important midline.

Meeting the Primal Midline

The primal midline is a constantly uprising midline apparent in the bioelectric torus-shaped field we sense at a long-tide level of perception. It differs from the midline of

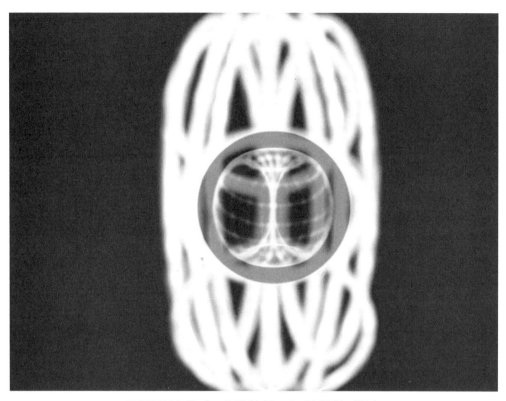

FIGURE 32: Bioelectric Field (Torus) with Field of Light

what we call the quantum field, or field of light, also established in relation to the individual at conception. The quantum midline can be perceived as running straight down the center of the physical body from the crown of the head to the center of the perineum. This quantum field is universal and essentially unaffected by the conditions of life. The very slow, very constant inhalations and exhalations of long tide widen out from and return in to this quantum midline. In contrast, the primal midline and its bioelectric torus manifest as a universal phenomenon, as well as relating to the individual and guiding individual development in the embryo and throughout life. Rather than presenting as a straight, unmodified line of light, like the quantum midline, the primal midline curves forward in relation to the folding of the embryo in the fourth week after conception. It therefore runs through the base of the skull and then forward and out through the center of the forehead, often referred to as the third-eye region.

Several researchers have noticed the universality of similar energetic fields and forces organizing everything in nature. For example, Austrian "water wizard" Viktor Schauberger noted that everything in nature, including water, is organized within energetic spirals or vortices, torus-shaped fields, each with a central midline or axis of stillness. Interestingly, in his native German language, the word for our boney midline, the spinal column, is *Wirbelsaule,* apparently actually meaning "spiral column"![132] As in Craniosacral Biodynamics, Schauberger perceived that "creative energy moves spirally in the form of a vortex. The creative process takes place as the energy containing the blueprint of what is being created moves in whatever way it needs to in order to create the system it wishes. It draws down matter as a mirror image of the idea or blueprint."[133] He saw the vortex as "the key to creative evolution … a window between different qualities or levels of energy."[134] This resonates with Sutherland's "transmutation," or change in state, of the Breath of Life into physical form. We might consider this transmutation as transference of vital information from the Breath of Life down into the cells.

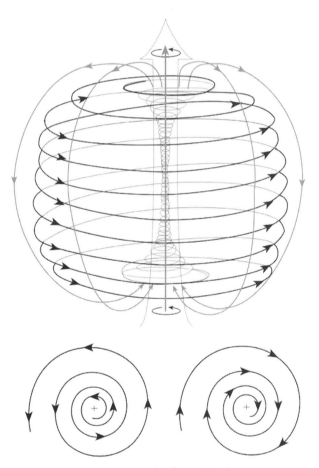

FIGURE 33: Schauberger Spiral
From Franklyn Sills, *Foundations in Craniosacral Biodynamics: The Breath of Life and Fundamental Skills, Vol. 1* (Berkeley, CA: North Atlantic Books, 2011), 23. Thanks to illustrator Dominique DeGranges.

Like all things in nature, we humans are organized within energetic fields. Medical science researcher Arthur Winfree was studying the heart in health and disease when he discovered energetic fields around the heart.[135] These seemed to be affected in heart arrhythmias, as well as being important in the formation of proteins and hormones and in biochemical processes like chemical bonding. Both Schauberger and Winfree described movement rising up the center or midline of a torus-shaped energetic field. This is how the primal midline is often perceived. Based on its constantly rising nature, as well as its embryological significance, we also refer to this midline as the "embryological arising."

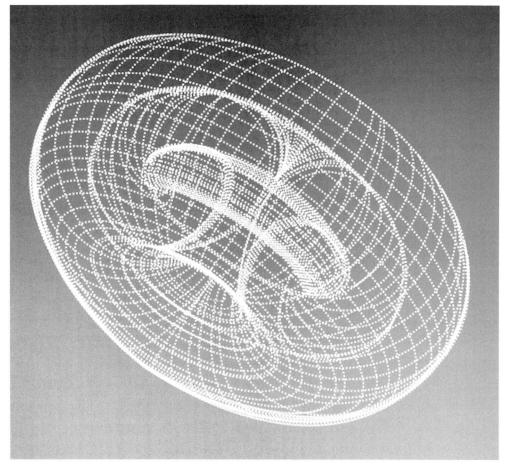

FIGURE 34: Winfree Scroll Ring

The Torus in Three-Dimensional Space, from Franklyn Sills, *Foundations in Craniosacral Biodynamics: The Breath of Life and Fundamental Skills, Vol. 1* (Berkeley, CA: North Atlantic Books, 2011), 290; based on Arthur T. Winfree, *When Time Breaks Down: The Three-Dimensional Dynamics of Electrochemical Waves and Cardiac Arrhythmias* (Princeton, NJ: Princeton University Press, 1987), 214. Thanks to illustrator Dominique DeGranges.

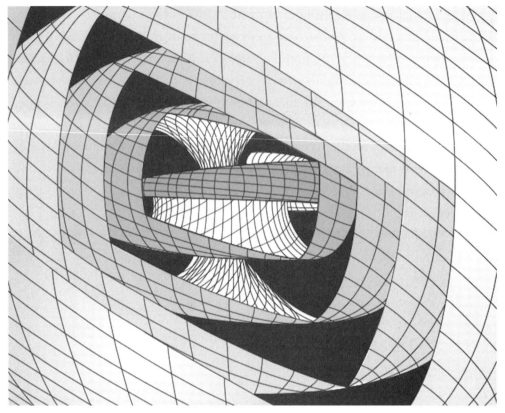

FIGURE 35: Fields within Fields: A View inside Winfree Scroll Rings to the Organizing Center Space is enfolded in order to generate form, from Franklyn Sills, *Foundations in Craniosacral Biodynamics: The Breath of Life and Fundamental Skills, Vol. 1* (Berkeley, CA: North Atlantic Books, 2011), 291; based on Arthur T. Winfree, *When Time Breaks Down: The Three-Dimensional Dynamics of Electrochemical Waves and Cardiac Arrhythmias* (Princeton, NJ: Princeton University Press, 1987), 215. Thanks to illustrator Dominique DeGranges.

An Embryo within Us

The bioenergetic torus and its ever-arising midline apparently guide the embryo in its formation, resonant with how all aspects of nature are organized. As mentioned earlier, scientists recently observing frog embryos were surprised to witness aspects of the embryo, like its face and eyes, forming first in a bioelectric field, and then, through exchange with this field, manifesting physically in the cells and tissues.[136] Watching the video on YouTube, you can also see what appears to be an energetic midline rising up the forming body of the frog embryo, followed by appearance of a physical midline.

The Breath of Life steps down into physical form, both in us and in other aspects of nature. An energetic blueprint apparently informs us, as indicated by Schauberger.

In this transmutation process, we coalesce into form, becoming increasingly physical. When we deepen into a long-tide level of perception, we seem to be accessing subtle rhythmic phenomena underlying our physical form. Within these bioenergetic fields of support and guidance, the tiny embryo takes form. The very first expression of physical form in the embryo is a line, called the primitive streak, arising along the center of what will become its backside. For the first two weeks after conception, the new being is busy first finding a home, a place to implant in the uterine wall to ensure it has a source of nourishment. Further supporting its essential need for food, as well as removal of waste products, the embryo then intelligently constructs what develops into the placenta and umbilical cord. Once this important infrastructure is established, it begins building its body, starting with the primitive streak. Until this line appears fourteen days after conception, the embryo is essentially an undifferentiated mass of cells. Let's examine this process in a bit more detail.

Embryo development begins with cell division of the original fertilized egg, or zygote, soon after conception. As the cells divide and multiply, the embryo looks like

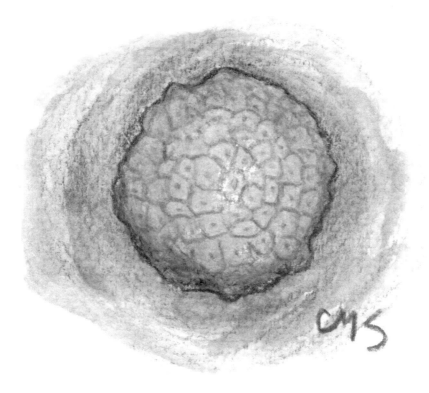

FIGURE 36: Embryo as Ball of Cells

a ball of cells. Some of the cells develop into precursors of the umbilical cord and placenta. In the first week or so after implantation, the embryo intelligently establishes this source of nourishment first, laying a supportive ground for developing the remaining cells, aligned as two simple layers—the hypoblast and epiblast—into what we recognize as the baby's body. In figure 37, we see that the bilaminar (two-layered) disc of the embryo itself is but a tiny portion of the whole structure it has created inside the wall of the mother's womb.

Once the essential infrastructure has been established, the first major change in appearance in the clump of cells to become the main body of the embryo is the sudden emergence of a midline, the primitive streak. The primitive streak arises within the primal midline fourteen days after conception as cells are seemingly drawn upward through the center of the embryo by the pull of the constantly arising primal midline. As it rises, a third layer of cells is created between the original two layers of bilaminar

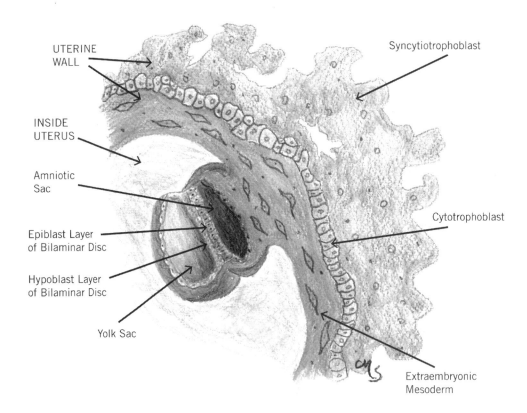

FIGURE 37: Early Bilaminar Embryo within Sacs
Based on T. W. Sadler, *Langman's Medical Embryology,* 11th ed., International ed.
(London: Lippincott Williams & Wilkins, 2010), 56, fig. 1.

disc, which now becomes a trilaminar (three-layered) disc. The embryo begins to be more than two-dimensional, having a bit of substance filling the sandwich of its outer layers. At this point, it has three layers you probably learned about in biology classes. They are commonly known as the ectoderm, endoderm, and mesoderm. The embryo then takes another important step toward physical manifestation as the notochord soon follows the primitive streak in its course up the midline. The relatively condensed embryonic tissue of the notochord then serves as a fulcrum, or organizing central space of stillness, around which the embryo forms. The bodies of the vertebrae and intervertebral discs between them literally form around the notochord. Figure 38 depicts this mysterious arising of the midline in the early embryo. To understand the phenomenon better, I recommend watching a YouTube video of a frog embryo developing at this state at https://www.youtube.com/watch?v=IkqBzEzuIc4 (one of the inspirations for

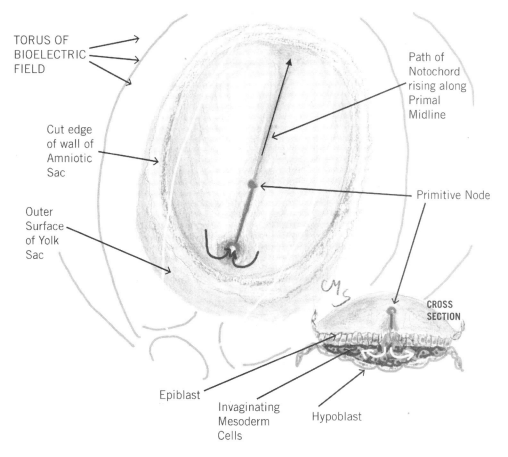

TORUS OF BIOELECTRIC FIELD

Path of Notochord rising along Primal Midline

Cut edge of wall of Amniotic Sac

Primitive Node

Outer Surface of Yolk Sac

CROSS SECTION

Epiblast

Invaginating Mesoderm Cells

Hypoblast

FIGURE 38: Primitive Streak and Notochord Rising up the Primal Midline within the Torus
Illustrations inspired by https://www.youtube.com/watch?v=IkqBzEzuIc4 and Sadler, 2010, p. 57.

the illustration). There are also excellent animations of this entire process on You-Tube, which can help you understand the changes involved (e.g., https://youtu.be /iHmBIJs77ZQ).

In Craniosacral Biodynamics, we sense the primal midline running up through the centers of the vertebral bodies and intervertebral discs along the path of the notochord. While most of the notochord does not persist after the fetus develops, the organizing influence of primal midline remains. We sense this as an energetic arising. In a healthy system, we can sense the primal midline rising from the coccyx and sacrum all the way up through the base of the occiput, the body of the sphenoid and the ethmoid bone, all formed like the vertebrae in relation to the path of the notochord and its energetic guide, the primal midline.

As the embryo continues to develop, all the body's tissues form in relation to the notochord. It is easy to see the bodies of the vertebrae clearly form around this organizing fulcrum in their center. Along with other connective tissues in the body, the

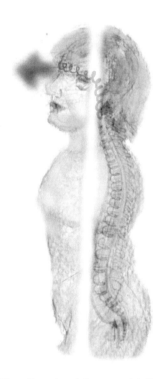

FIGURE 39: Primal and Quantum Midlines

spine forms from coalesced embryonic tissue called somites, which present as bumps on either side of the notochord midline.

This is a process of differentiation. As pointed out by embryologist Jaap van der Wal, the embryo is "falling apart into separate body parts," beginning, and always maintaining itself as a whole.[137] The original clump of cells begins to differentiate with the first appearance of the primitive streak. Up to this point, all of the cells of the embryo are basically the same. Looking at the embryo, we cannot before this point identify back, front, top, bottom, left, or right. With the appearance of the primitive streak, however, this changes. The streak, like the primal midline guiding it, rises up from the tail end of the clump of cells. We can then see where the tail and head ends are. We also know that the streak presents on what will become the dorsal or backside of the embryo. Front and back are now differentiated, also enabling us to recognize the left and right sides. The embryo has begun falling into its parts, following the arising of the primal midline. The notochord then continues up the midline where the primitive streak stops. The streak appears to recede as the embryo grows longer, and eventually

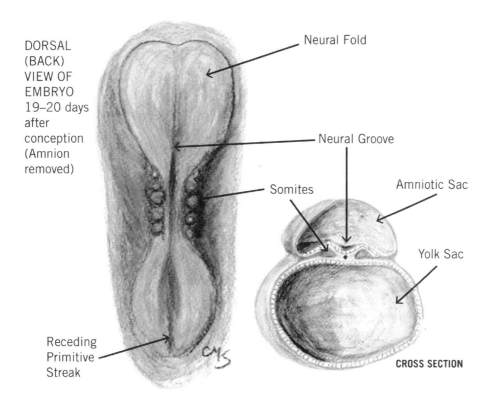

DORSAL (BACK) VIEW OF EMBRYO 19–20 days after conception (Amnion removed)

Neural Fold

Neural Groove

Somites

Amniotic Sac

Yolk Sac

Receding Primitive Streak

CROSS SECTION

FIGURE 40: Somites Forming around Notochord

only the notochord remains, deeper under the ectoderm. We can consider this first coalescing of embryonic fluid tissue as representative of the bioelectric torus and its primal midline. This is a wonderful depiction of the transmutation from a bioelectric to a fluid-cellular-tissue level of expression!

While you may or may not be as fascinated as I am by embryological development, it is highly relevant to our work with Craniosacral Biodynamics. Just as the little embryo follows the unseen but reliable guidance of the bioelectric field and its primal midline, so do we throughout our lives. In biodynamic session work, it is not unusual as the inherent treatment plan unfolds to perceive this powerful midline as an organizing influence in the reorganization process. Once an inertial fulcrum has resolved, the entire system can shift, no longer needing to organize in relation to this inertial event. Not only do we sense changes, like softening, spreading, and greater coherence and ease of motion in the local area affected by the now-resolved inertial fulcrum, but we also sense the entire system reorganizing. In this process, it is often as if the client has returned to a relatively fluid, undifferentiated embryonic state, and can orient again to the primal midline.

It is important to understand that the primal midline and bioelectric field represent universal biodynamic forces. The system strives to stay oriented to the health-supporting guidance of these forces. Where conditional forces have affected the system, however, the tissue's ability to orient to the primal midline may be occluded by the influence of inertial fulcrums containing the conditional forces. As a fulcrum is resolved, and the conditional forces it has been holding are discharged, the potency that has been containing them becomes available for other life-supporting functions. The ability to access the original biodynamic forces is re-established.

I find it helpful here to consider the teachings of Emilie Conrad, founder of Continuum Movement. In her almost fifty years of inquiring into our fluid nature through movement and awareness, Conrad realized that our tissues change in relation to their context. She identified what she called "three tissue anatomies."[138] In our everyday fetch wood–carry water state, we tend to be sped up, task-focused, and often overwhelmed. Our tissues, like our attention, become more dense and narrow. If we try to stretch or exercise in this state, we can easily become injured as our tight tissues lose flexibility and resilience. Conrad called this the cultural anatomy, influenced as it is by our cultural context. As we slow down in Continuum practice, we begin to melt. Our tissues literally become softer and more fluid, and begin to spread. We begin to enter what Conrad called the primordial anatomy. Here, we become more like the little embryo, less differentiated, with more sense of wholeness and often having an awareness of midline. To me, this is a description of the fluid body or field in Craniosacral Biodynamics, as we deepen under the CRI, which relates to the cultural anatomy.

As we continue to slow down and deepen further in Continuum, we experience the cosmic anatomy. Similar to long tide, in this state we have more of a sense of airy space and ether. We often feel as if we are suspended in the cosmos, an immensely supportive energetic field. Remember that the torus is universal in nature. It is seen everywhere in the cosmos. I heard Conrad say many times, "The cosmos is spiraled water. The embryo is spiraled water." In a more watery state, the fluid of the embryo and the cosmos directly communicate through resonance. As we slow down and melt, we can re-enter that state of resonant relationship with that which is beyond us. In biodynamic terms, this is a more direct connection with the Breath of Life, as it steps down into the long tide and the bioelectric field. Suspended in this supportive field, we can re-form ourselves. Our tissues can reshape themselves in relation to this relatively unconditioned context.

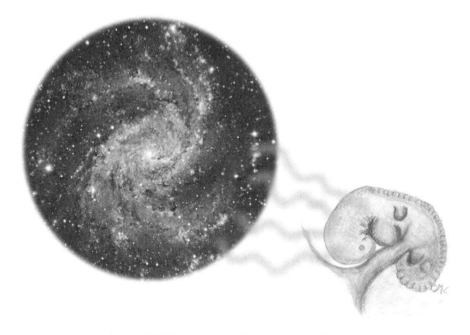

FIGURE 41: Embryo Resonating with Cosmos
Spiral Galaxy credit NGC 6946 (HST, Subaru); Credit: NASA, ESA, STScI, R. Gendler, and the Subaru Telescope (NAOJ); http://hubblesite.org/image/3678/gallery; Embryo illustration inspired by A. Grey, *Transfigurations* (Rochester, VT: Inner Traditions, 2001), 77.

Journeying Beyond Genetics

We can understand this renewal more fully by again returning to our small but important teacher, the embryo. Despite what you may have learned in biology classes, in the first few weeks of life, development is not directed by genes.

The important embryologist Erich Blechschmidt proposed that how embryological cells develop is determined by their position. He wrote, "For any ensemble of cells, positional development determines development of their form, and this, in turn, determines their structural development."[139] Although all cells have the same genes, their positional context affects which genes are turned on at any particular time.

Cell biologist Bruce Lipton enlarges this view in his explanation of how the pregnant woman's perception of her environment as either safe and nurturing or hostile affects which genes are turned on during development of her baby.[140] In this way, the baby growing within the context of how the mother perceives her environment is being prepared to best meet and survive in the environment it is to be born into. Lipton was an early proponent of what has developed into the important field of epigenetics.

Epigenetics literally means "over, outside, or around genetics." To me, this is a perfect way to refer to biodynamic forces! We might say genetics operate within the fields within fields of support and guidance provided by the step-downs of the Breath of Life. I appreciate that, in the modern field of embryology, fields are recognized as influencing development. For example, to continue quoting Blechschmidt, "The metabolic processes occurring in cells or their ensembles not only have a chemical significance, but also always display accompanying physical and special (morphological) characteristics. Accordingly, one can think of cellular ensembles and organs respectively as locally modified force fields. Here we mean fields that are everywhere impregnated with submicroscopic particles moving in an ordered manner."[141]

Morphology refers to the shaping of the embryo. The appearance of the primitive streak and notochord are the beginning of the embryo's change of shape from a living but undifferentiated ball of cells into a creature characterized by different parts, a spherical shape with a line running through it. I see this as an example of Blechschmidt's "locally modified force field." We have the bioenergetic force field of the torus and its primal midline guiding this process. The cells close to the primal midline are directly ordered by it, following it up toward what will become the cranial end of the embryo.

In session work, we can again see changes in shape. Inertial patterns may present as shapes within the cellular-tissue field of the client. As the inertial fulcrum organizing the pattern is resolved, the patterned shape shifts. There is a reordering in relation to the primal midline. The client's shape may literally present as more symmetrical than it was prior to the treatment. This represents a return to the original embryological intention.

In the first few weeks after conception, we all look the same. Our individual genes have not yet been ignited. We all have a primitive streak and notochord along the midline. We all look relatively symmetrical, being mostly midline, until we begin to sprout little arm and leg buds and our organs begin to take shape, starting with the heart in the fourth week after conception. Even the heart begins as a midline structure, developing at the cranial end of the embryo. During the fourth week as the developing nervous system grows over the heart, the embryo folds, bringing the heart to meet the energetic heart center. At this point, it miraculously begins beating, with another energetic ignition.

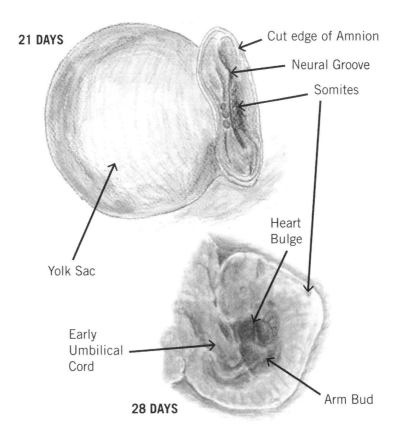

FIGURE 42: Embryo Folding
Illustration inspired by G.C. Schoenworlf, S. B. Bleyl, P. R. Brauer, and P. H. Francis-West *Larsen's Embryology, 4th ed.* (London: Churchill Livingstone, 2009), 109; and A. Grey, *Transfigurations* (Rochester, VT: Inner Traditions, 2001), 77.

It is not unusual during the reorganization phase of a session to perceive not only the primal midline lighting up as a guiding force, but also to feel like we are holding a little embryo. Often, we sense an embryonic folding, as if the client were revisiting this momentous embryological event. During this reordering process, I often have a sense of my own heart warming and softening, as if I am actually holding a little one. I may even have an image, or felt sense, of having a little embryo in my hands. I feel my heart touched even as I write this. Do you feel it as you read these words?

Touching the Heart of the Embryo

The experience of folding is associated with a powerful ignition of the first organ to come online, the heart. In the embryo, this occurs in the fourth week after conception. According to prenatal and birth psychology pioneer William Emerson, this is also the time of discovery, when the pregnancy tends to be confirmed.[142] While the news of being pregnant may be completely celebrated by the expectant parents, most often it is accompanied by at least some degree of ambivalence. Even couples longing to conceive a child may be surprised or taken off guard when it happens. It is not unusual for parents to feel they aren't ready, that the time isn't quite right. The pregnancy may even be very unwelcome news, triggering extreme fear, anxiety, anger, and other challenging emotions for the mother or both parents.

The little one floating inside is affected by the parents' reaction to discovering its existence. Appropriately, the tiny being may feel safe and secure if the parents celebrate but fear for its life if it is unwanted. If the parents consider abortion, survival is obviously in question. Adoption may also be terrifying for the little one, who physiologically depends on maternal acceptance. Rejection or abandonment biologically spells danger for the completely dependent baby. Regardless of your opinions about the possibility of remembering such early events, there is now ample evidence that individuals are powerfully affected by their earliest prenatal experiences and tend to live their lives accordingly. If you have trouble with this concept, just consider for a moment how even single-celled creatures react to danger by withdrawing. If you think cells can't remember, consider that our health depends on cells in our immune system being able to remember and identify danger. It is not too much of a stretch to understand that a tiny embryo, much more complex by the fourth week than a unicellular organism, can react to a sense of danger or the maternal hormones involved with extreme emotions.

These reactions, even while usually not based on conscious experience, are as relevant to our work as the embryological ignitions enabling them. In fact, ignition of the heart may be dampened in challenging or dangerous conditions. Similarly, ignition at conception may be less full than is potentially possible when conception occurs in unsupportive conditions. In Craniosacral Biodynamics, we work directly with augmenting these ignitions in our clients when appropriate. Where ignition has been less than fully manifested in the embryo, we may perceive sluggishness in the client's system, which may be accompanied by varying symptoms. Working with ignition processes can be very supportive.

Having awareness of the psychological and emotional territory that may relate to this time can be helpful in holding a client, as these early experiential memories may surface during session work. In the next chapter, we discuss working with trauma in biodynamic sessions, but for now it is important to have awareness that these early, even prenatal, territories can arise. We don't want to go looking for them or expecting them, as this introduces an external force into the system. If they do arise, however, it is useful to be able to recognize and meet them. Just energetically acknowledging what is presenting may be healing for a client whose very existence was not welcomed or appreciated as an embryo.

Holding the client as suspended within the bioelectric torus with its primal midline as guidance can facilitate profound healing on many levels. Inertial fulcrums can be resolved. The entire system can reorganize in relation to the biodynamic forces represented by the primal midline. Early psychological wounding may also heal within the fields within fields of support in the session, as cells, physiology, and structure all return to greater alignment with an original embryological intention.

I like to think of what occurs here as returning to our original embryological potential. When we consider, as we have in this chapter, our earliest beginnings, we can marvel at the incredible potential held within a single cell at conception. Is it not a miracle that each of us folds and unfolds into this recognizable human form from such humble, tiny beginnings! One fertilized egg cell has the potential to develop into this magnificent human form, apparently following instructions of an invisible, energetic blueprint.

As life happens, and conditions have their effects, we may stray from our original potential. In biodynamic sessions, we have the ability to return to the potential of our earliest beginnings. As we settle under our everyday speed, rest into the safety of our relational field, potency as an ever-ready harbinger of potential is able to do its work to clear the clouds and reveal once again the sunny clarity of our being. The Breath of Life can breathe through us with greater ease and we remember, our cells and tissues remember, who we truly are.

Primal Midline Experiential

This guided exploration is designed to introduce you to the primal midline within your own body. You may want to record these instructions in your own voice and play them back to yourself to enable you to focus more internally through this exploration. (A recording is available at www.birthingyourlife.org/the-breath-of-life-book/.) This experiential involves making sounds into your primal midline, inspired by Continuum, to enhance your ability to sense your midline. Take a moment before settling into your body to acquaint yourself with the path of the primal midline, as viewed in in figure 43 below.

As we have before, take some time to find a comfortable seated position, being curious in the process about the sensations informing you. What tells you that you are comfortable or not? Do you have a sense of your breath? Can you sense your body where it makes contact with what you are sitting on? What is the quality of that contact? Do you feel like you are resting into the support of gravity, hovering above it, resisting it, or a different kind of relationship with the support of the earth under you? How is it to inquire into your sensations in this way?

Taking note of any sense of settling, softening, melting, or slowing down, you may begin to have more of a sense of wholeness and perhaps of Primary Respiration. What speaks to you of midline as you settle more deeply?

Once you have a sense of your breath and ground, your physical body, allow your field of perception to begin to widen out beyond the boundaries of your skin while staying grounded. Let yourself orient to any sense of fluidity and perhaps mid-tide, a sense of building, filling, surging up midline, widening out from midline, then narrowing back in toward it and down toward the earth in two to three cycles per minute. Allow yourself to rest in mid-tide, being curious about any sense of potency, aliveness, or life energy here.

After some time orienting to mid-tide, allow your awareness to begin to widen further, perhaps first to include the whole room, then gradually widening out toward the horizon in all directions, but not so far that you lose your sense of yourself and your midline. Stay with the midline fulcrum and widen from there, perhaps thinking of widening out from your

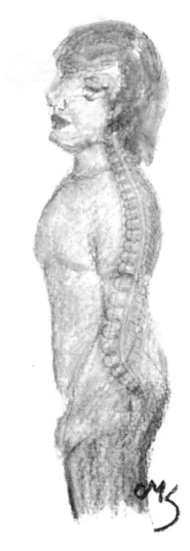

FIGURE 43: Primal Midline Rising through Vertebrae

belly, rather than from your head to help with staying grounded. Allow yourself to rest, to be in this wider field of perception. You may have a sense of long tide drawing your awareness in toward midline or out toward the horizon in very slow cycles, fifty seconds in each direction. There may be a sense of sparkly radiance. You may feel as if you are suspended within a vast energetic field.

Once you have a sense of the support of this vastness, allow yourself to include a sense of primal midline. This is the path of the notochord up through the bodies of the vertebrae, at the front of the spine. It may feel almost halfway between the back and front of your body.

Orient to any sense of arising here. It may feel like heat rising up, like wind or fire or even like air rising up a hot air shaft. Or you may sense it visually, like light rising up through the midline. Don't worry if you don't sense this right away. Just let yourself be curious as you rest within the wide field, with an awareness of the midline area of your body. With your wide field of perception, you may be aware of the midline as arising within a torus-shaped field around you.

Let's add a bit more input here to awaken awareness of this primal midline. I'd like to invite you to make a sound and visualize it rising up your midline. This is an "O" sound, like the letter "O." Make the sound as if you were humming the O. Take an easy, relatively deep, full breath in, if possible with your mouth closed. Then, on the exhale, allow the O to gently, slowly resonate in your tissues. Let yourself be curious about what you sense as you make the O sound. When you are at the end of your out breath, without effort, take another easy breath in and make another O. As you make the O sound, imagine, sense, visualize moving up from the tailbone through the lower spine, thoracic vertebrae, the cervical vertebrae, and then through the base of the skull and forward to the center of your forehead, between your eyes, the space often associated with the third eye. Make as many Os as you need to reach the top. If you are familiar with the anatomy, think of passing through the centers of the vertebral bodies, then through the base of the occiput, body of the sphenoid, and to the ethmoid bone. Some people have a sense of this rising midline spraying out through the ethmoid/third-eye area as a "fountain spray of life," named by Randolph Stone, osteopath and founder of Polarity Therapy.[143]

Take your time doing the Os into this midline. I like to think of this kind of sounding, which comes from Continuum, as offering the vibration of the sound to the tissues. Can you sense the vibration in the spine or anywhere else in your body? Are there places along the midline where it is easier to sense than others? Or where there seems to be a blockage or density? Feel free to offer extra Os to such areas. There are probably inertial fulcrums in these areas. I find the Os support the potency in doing its work as needed, and you may find the density softening and more sense of energy moving through these areas.

Once you have reached the top of the midline, the forehead, with your Os, take some time in what we call "open attention" in Continuum. This is a time of simply listening. You have offered a gift to your tissues. Now, let yourself be curious about how your tissues respond, receive, and integrate. What do you sense? How is your breath? What sensations are you aware of? Do you sense anything different in your back, along your midline, or anywhere else in your body? Perhaps you have a sense of movement spontaneously arising. If you are comfortable doing so, allow this movement. Often there will be a sense of fluid movement, expressing as slow pulsations, waves, or spirals. This is a response to the sound. It is as if you have stirred the waters of your body with the vibration of the Os. The movement is the rippling of the water in response. Where it ripples freely, there is more fluidity. Like water in a river, the ripples may run into denser areas, like rocks in the river. Notice how the movement splashes up against these denser areas. It can begin to help loosen them.

When you are satisfied with your exploration, feel free to repeat the Os if you want to. When you are done with your open attention, allow yourself to again rest into a sense of suspension within a wide field, taking note of any sense of midline. What speaks to you of midline now?

Take some time to be with your experience, perhaps sensing mid-tide and fluidity, then returning to a sense of your physical body, breath, and ground. Let your body move any way that feels good to you. Gently bring your awareness back to the room, opening your eyes, looking around to orient yourself. You may want to take some time to take some notes about your experience.

7

Past into Present

Introduction to Working with Trauma Arising in Biodynamic Sessions

While trauma can be hell on earth, trauma resolved is a gift from the gods—a heroic journey that belongs to each of us.
—PETER LEVINE[144]

Have you ever had one of those days when you start out feeling like life is your oyster, but then there's no hot water for the shower? You can't find the shirt you were going to wear. Then you spill your morning coffee, staining your shirt, and don't really have time to change it. You are finally finished with breakfast and getting dressed for the second time when you receive a message informing you that someone close to you has just become very ill or their husband left them for another woman or some other tragedy occurred, and they really need your support. The day continues in this vein and at some point you feel like you can't take anymore.

I'm sorry to start this chapter on such a depressing note, but when people have experienced overwhelming trauma, every day can feel this difficult. Often, those with trauma in their history start their days already depressed and overwhelmed, rather than feeling the world is theirs for the taking. They may carry their unresolved trauma as chronic pain, ongoing depression, anxiety, or other body-mind disturbances.[145] It is common for Craniosacral Therapy to touch upon old traumas stored in the body-mind, and clients often come to us because of them.

Trauma is not just physical. Our body-minds function as one unit. We now know that trauma, or overwhelming experiences, affects how our nervous system functions. Physical trauma can leave the nervous system overstimulated, resulting in chronic pain, immune problems and psychological issues like depression.[146] It is common for people to develop post-traumatic stress disorder (PTSD) following orthopedic surgery, cancer treatment, or a stay in intensive care.[147]

Clients coming to us with physical problems often have psychological issues accompanying their physical symptoms. There may be unresolved emotional trauma associated with or underlying the physical concerns. These may arise unexpectedly during the sessions. This chapter introduces this important territory, along with some helpful ways to meet trauma when it arises in session work. Clients also come to Craniosacral Therapy sessions seeking support in becoming calmer, reducing anxiety and depression, and easing insomnia. Children are brought to address issues with attention, learning, and behavior. Babies are treated when they cry inconsolably, have colic or other digestive problems, or had a difficult birth. All of these can relate to trauma. To support us recognizing and addressing the emergence of trauma in biodynamic session work, we'll first consider trauma in general.

What Is Trauma?

Our understanding of trauma has evolved dramatically in recent years. Not long ago, people suffering the ongoing effects of an overwhelming experience, like war or rape, were expected to go on to perform in their lives as if nothing had happened. Trauma specialists now recognize that the neurobiology of trauma can interfere with a person's ability to function in everyday life. A traumatized person may experience the present moment as if the trauma were happening here and now. Peter Levine, founder of Somatic Experiencing, offers a modern definition of trauma:

> Trauma is a form of implicit memory that is profoundly unconscious, and forms the basis for the imprint trauma leaves on the body/mind. The bodies of traumatized people portray "snapshots" of their unsuccessful attempts to defend themselves in the face of threat and injury ... Trauma is fundamentally a highly activated incomplete biological response to threat, frozen in time.[148]

It can be helpful to take some time to define the word *trauma,* as it is used in many ways, even within the fields of psychology and medicine. For example, medical trauma refers to physical injuries or conditions that have presented suddenly and require immediate medical attention. In everyday life, we tend to use the word *trauma* to refer to a particularly stressful event. The experience of trauma, however, varies between individuals. What is traumatizing for one may be just another moment for someone else.

Trauma involves a sense of being overwhelmed by the given circumstance or event. This relates to how resourced we are when the event occurs. For instance, if you have had a good night's sleep, are generally healthy, and feel good about yourself, your life, and your relationships, you are less likely to be overwhelmed than if you haven't slept well in a month, are just getting over the flu, have just had a relationship end, have lost a job, or had a new baby. All of these things are stressful.

The term *stress* was coined by researcher Hans Selye, who first described the stress response in 1936. He defined stress as "the non-specific response of the body to any demand for change."[149] Selye noted that the first response to stress is alarm, followed by fight-or-flight, and then adaptation. Adaptation uses energy, thus depleting our resources. If we don't replenish them, we become exhausted and less able to deal with stress. Some stress is good for us. Without resistance or challenge, there is no learning or development. Each step of our embryological development is an expression of the embryo meeting the challenges and conditions of its current environment.[150, 151, 152] This is inherently stressful, but hopefully not overwhelmingly so. For example, the embryo implants in the uterine wall when its growth has reached a point that it requires a new external source of nourishment. If implantation does not happen easily, it becomes urgent, as the embryo is in danger of starvation. Implantation may then become traumatic. It is not uncommon for people in prenatal therapy to remember or feel as if they are implanting and to describe the challenges involved. Where it has been traumatic, they may have struggled throughout life to find a place to settle and feel at home, to feel welcomed and well-nourished. If implantation or other stages of development are well-supported and relatively easy, they lay a foundation for relative ease and stability upon which we build our lives.

I am reminded of the American Sign Language sign for spring, which is a hand pushing through the fist of the other hand to rise up like a young plant. Plants require some resistance from the earth in order to push their heads up through it. You may have patted the earth down after planting a seed to provide the necessary resistance. Similarly, natural vaginal birth provides the baby with useful resistance, which serves as a massage and organizing influence for the whole body and its physiology. Babies born by cesarean section who do not push their way out of the womb tend to suffer breathing and immune problems. When the resistance within the birth canal is too much, however, it can become traumatizing. The baby is overwhelmed, and often the mother is too. Their resources are drained. Other stressors often come into the picture during birth, such as ongoing noise and other stimulation from multiple birth attendants and hospital activities. Babies traumatized at birth often come for Craniosacral Therapy. If they are not brought when they are little, they may find their way to our treatment rooms years later, not consciously remembering their birth journey or aware of its profound effects on every aspect of their lives.

The transfer to a hospital is in itself stressful, even if it has been planned and the parents feel safer being in a hospital. Being removed from the familiar, usually relatively quiet environment of home and taken to the sterile hospital, usually with some

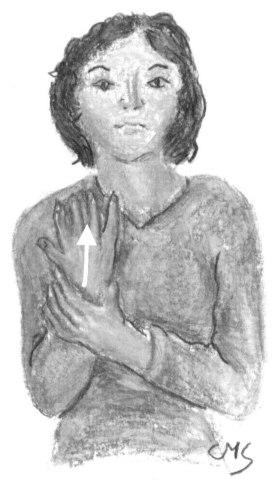

FIGURE 44: American Sign Language Sign "Spring"

degree of anxiety and hastiness, requires the mother to adapt to new surroundings (and baby to adjust to Mom's adaptations). This process can deplete her of energy needed for labor. Usually, due to the release of stress hormones, labor slows down or stops during the trip to hospital.[153] This often leads to medical interventions, which, while possibly helpful, add to the stress. They are unnatural experiences that need to be adapted to by both mother and baby. As Jean Liedloff notes in her book *The Continuum Concept*, millions of years have prepared us for natural birth.[154]

Liedloff describes the stressful effects of not meeting "the inherent expectations of [our] species" based on our evolutionary history.[155] She sees "change," unlike evolution, as "replac[ing] a piece of well-integrated behavior with one that is not. It replaces what is complex and adapted with what is simpler and less adapted. As a consequence, change places a strain on the equilibrium of all the intricately related factors inside and outside the system."[156] Our modern medical birth practices are an example of this kind of disruptive change, initiated by intellect, without fully understanding or respecting what evolution had already established.

Medicalized birth, like other medical procedures, tends to involve a sense of urgency and speed. These also add to the stress, as there is often not enough time given to adapt to each new intervention or change. This is one way in which birth, a very natural and potentially joyful event, can become overly stressful and, therefore, traumatic. In one research study, four out of five birthing women described their birth as traumatic. One in ten women was diagnosed with PTSD after giving birth.[157]

Remember that the experience of trauma relates to the degree of resource or overwhelm. I suggest practicing remembering your resources while reading this chapter, since we have all been born and we have all experienced various traumatizing events. Reorienting to resource, what supports you, can help balance any tendency to have your own stress or trauma responses activated as you read. One reason to include a chapter on trauma in this introductory book is that we as practitioners need to be able to meet our clients from a place of resource rather than from our own trauma reactions. Awareness can support this skill. *In this moment, can you sense your breath? Can you feel your feet or seat making contact with the floor or chair, sensing the support of gravity under you? Can you think of other things that are supportive for you and enable you to rest and be as you read?*

While we tend to think of traumas as being dramatic, life-threatening events, even simple daily activities can become traumatizing when resources are low. I had a powerful demonstration of this in my own life when I moved from Boulder, Colorado, to

Santa Barbara, California, in 2001, the week before my doctoral dissertation was due. The timing had just worked out that way, as I needed to be in Santa Barbara in time to start teaching at the Santa Barbara Graduate Institute. Needless to say, my first week in my new home was stressful! Instead of finding furniture, decorating, and settling in, I got right to work editing my final documents for my PhD. The day they were due was September 11. That morning, I was making my final revisions when my new roommate knocked on my door. I tried to ignore her and keep working, as I just had a few more hours before I needed to take the documents to the post office. "No!" she insisted. "This is important!" Of course, it was important. Not only was the entire country traumatized by the attack on the Twin Towers in New York, but all delivery services were frozen. I could not send my documents even though they were ready to go!

This was my landing in California. Things didn't get much better, although I was able after a few days to send in my final documents and the readers were understanding of my predicament. Shortly after moving to Santa Barbara, I discovered that the three jobs I had been promised had all fallen through! I had no income except a minimal teaching fee. I was in a new town and state I knew very little about. I was exhausted from years of putting every moment and penny into my doctoral studies, as well as moving across the country, and I had left my familiar life and community behind in Colorado. In this resource-drained condition, I sometimes found I could not handle going into a store to buy things. It was all too new, too much. I would stand at the door of the shop and feel I just could not do it. I could not go through that door and adapt to one more new experience. A few months later, when I had recovered, I noticed how it was not only easy to go into new shops, but I actually enjoyed and thrived on the experience. Having adequate energy and resources to adapt, I could meet the world again. I had returned to my usual curious self.

In my state of exhaustion, going into a new store was traumatizing. Overwhelming trauma has this same effect. It is too much for the person to deal with at the time. Adaptation is too much. In biodynamic terms, we describe the potency, or life energy, as being in its protective function. It is locked up in centering or containing inertial forces held in the system. If there is not enough potency available, a new force becomes difficult to meet. Its effects overwhelm the system, and we experience trauma.

One of the effects of trauma is that we become less resilient in our responses to stress. When the potency centers inertial forces, the body tends to hold certain postures, with chronic areas of holding or tension. The tissues tighten as a result of the potency coalescing. When faced with further stress, we tend to tighten further into these patterns. Consider how it is to walk if you have injured a hip, knee, or ankle, or are stiff due to arthritis. You may be able to walk, but if you unexpectedly step on uneven ground, your body stiffens in its usual pattern, rather than adjusting to the change. You experience familiar pain rather than being able to resiliently adjust to the changes in the surface. Trauma tends to affect our responses to life in a similar way. For example, a child who has grown up in a violent household, observing his mother repeatedly beaten up by his father, will tend to encounter or enact violence in his relationships. Soldiers who have survived battle scenes where their friends have been killed are often changed when they return home, struggling with a violent temper and uncontrolled aggression. A person who has been frozen with fear or unable to move in a car accident may tend to freeze again in stressful situations.

The understanding of trauma has developed over the years to the point where the condition termed post-traumatic stress disorder (PTSD) has been added to the DSM-5 (*Diagnostic and Statistical Manual of Mental Disorders,* Fifth Edition), the bible of the American Psychiatric Association.

The criteria for diagnosis in this most recent edition of the DSM include a serious stressor: "The person was exposed to: death, threatened death, actual or threatened serious injury, or actual or threatened sexual violence." A major aspect of this syndrome is "intrusion symptoms," or the recurrence of memories of the traumatic event through repetitive play in children, nightmares, flashbacks, and intense distress and physiologic reactions to stimuli reminiscent of the trauma. These symptoms relate to the tendency of the body-mind to repeat what has occurred, in thoughts and emotions, as well as in tissue and nervous system patterning. There seems to be an ongoing seeking of resolution to experience that has not yet been fully digested or integrated. When these symptoms occur spontaneously, they can be frightening and disorienting. When they emerge within a safe, supportive, therapeutic relational field, they can begin to resolve with appropriate guidance. The rest of this chapter looks at how these issues may present in biodynamic sessions, and how their resolution can be facilitated in that context.

The Importance of Trauma Awareness in Craniosacral Biodynamics

When clients carry unresolved trauma, it may manifest in biodynamic sessions in different ways. First, we may become aware of issues with relational field settling. As indicated in earlier chapters, settling the relational field between client and practitioner is an essential first step in the inherent treatment plan. Without settling, the client's system remains oriented to defensive strategies. The potency is locked up in its protective function and is less available for healing. The holistic shift cannot occur, or does not deepen, until the person can begin to rest in the relationship with the practitioner.

For clients with unresolved trauma, the practitioner may represent an abusive or neglectful parent, teacher, doctor, or other authority figure from the past. Consider that even well-meaning doctors, birth attendants, nurses, and others within a medical setting may be perceived by the patient as insensitive, invasive, disrespectful, or otherwise overwhelming. This includes babies' experience before and during birth. Little ones in the womb have been known to bat away an amniocentesis needle,[158] and demonstrate reduced movement and heart rate variability following the puncture.[159] They have been observed contracting and withdrawing when mother decides to reach for a cigarette.[160] Babies react to a harsh and speedy environment and rough handling at birth with understandable screaming or withdrawal. Unable to process stimuli as quickly as adults do, they are easily overwhelmed in a hospital setting by the flurry of activity, lights, and noise, multiple staff and family members around them, medical poking and prodding, weighing and washing, and the common denial or lack of consideration for their feelings. These frequently traumatic first moments of life outside the womb can profoundly affect how the individual perceives and interacts with life thereafter.

Babies clearly demonstrate their memory of their birth in Craniosacral Therapy sessions. Whether their memories are acknowledged or not, their experience travels with them throughout their lives. It is not unusual in session work to have a client slip into an infantile state. It may feel as if we are holding a helpless little one. This regressive aspect of bodywork can be scary and disturbing if it stimulates traumatic memories. When these memories and the accompanying nervous system activations are met and held with gentle, reassuring awareness, the potential for healing and resolution is profound.

With unresolved trauma, clients' neurobiology is preoccupied with rerunning the challenge they encountered, forever seeking to avoid its recurrence. Ironically, it is not unusual for trauma victims to be drawn to situations that re-create the kind of trauma they are trying, often unconsciously, to avoid. Clients who have experienced abuse from parents or other authority figures in childhood may become frozen on the table with a practitioner. Unable to respond or to interact as an adult, or to set boundaries when contact feels invasive, such clients may experience inappropriate touch from a practitioner or be attracted to practitioners with unclear boundaries who take advantage of passive clients to seduce them or become romantic with them. Clients may arrive at a biodynamic session having had a previous experience like this. Clients come to us bringing their fears and expectations, as well as hopes.

As mentioned in an earlier chapter, I have had clients burst into tears when I ask how the contact is for them or express that it is important that they be comfortable. They tell me they are touched because no one has ever cared before. Others freeze on the table, unable to stay present with physical contact. They may be unable to express uncomfortable feelings, even if I ask them to let me know if anything isn't comfortable. This chapter includes an introduction to the underlying neurobiology of trauma responsible for these kinds of behaviors common in trauma that can interfere with relational field settling. The good news is that, when we are able to support clients in settling under these trauma reactions, essential healing can occur. These clients often experience dramatic shifts in their interpersonal relationships in life, as well as on the treatment table, as they learn to come into present time.

Trauma reactions may arise during sessions as specific patterns in the body are being worked with. It is common for clients to come to Craniosacral Therapy due to headaches or other symptoms relating to cranial issues. As we hold and work with the cranium, we may begin to feel like we are holding a tiny newborn head. When we consider the size of the human baby's head in relation to the pelvic opening it must pass through in vaginal birth, it is easy to understand the kind of forces the cranium must endure in this passage. Baby's skull bones are not fused at birth, being designed to be able to move and overlap with each other as necessary to negotiate the journey through the birth canal. When the baby can rest after birth, feeling safe on Mom's chest, hearing her heartbeat slowing down with relaxation after the stress of labor is complete, the tissues can reset themselves.

The cranial bones tend to naturally and spontaneously return to their prebirth alignment within a short time. Within a stressful environment, however, this relaxation is impeded. Babies may be removed from Mom and taken to intensive care or a newborn nursery. Even if they stay with their mothers, there may be speedy commotion all around them, with well-meaning professionals and relatives checking in on them. The stress hormones required for birth continue until things settle down. In this situation, the cranial bones may remain, at least to some degree, in their molded position. As the sutures, or spaces between the bones, close in during the following year or so, the bones become fixed in their compressed position.

Many of the issues we encounter in Craniosacral Therapy relate to this early birth trauma. Within the biodynamic session, the client's system is finally able to recognize safety and rest. The cranial patterns begin to resolve as the potency addresses the inertial forces holding them in place. During this process, the traumatic feelings and physiological reactions from the time of birth may present. The client may experience fear, anxiety, or anger that seems to just come up out of nowhere. Or there may be a sense of freezing, which may have been the infant's only way to deal with an overwhelming situation.

The following table lists some common ways to recognize when a client is in an adequately resourced state or is showing signs of trauma activation. Do any of these resonate with your experience?

TABLE 1

WHAT IS RESOURCE?	SIGNS OF RESOURCE:
• Supports us to be present, cope, reorient to health. • What is working in us now? • Outer resources help us connect with inner resources. • Who are the people (or animals) in your life who are resources for you? • Or fairies, goddesses, spiritual practices, or teachers? • Or favorite things, activities, clothes, jewelry, places, or images?	• Warmth • Expansion • Broader perspective • Relationship • Connectivity • Relaxation • Slowing down • Softening • Spreading • Movement organizes in a direction • Sense of fullness • Sense of wholeness
WHAT IS TRAUMA?	**SIGNS OF TRAUMA ACTIVATION:**
• When stress is too much for our current level of resource. • Our resources are exhausted. • Too many stresses at the same time. • New stress added to unresolved historical stresses. • Not enough resource to process, resolve, integrate the event.	• Speeding up • Holding breath/shallow breath • Trembling • Cold extremities • Intense heat • Dissociation • Numbing • Shock, overwhelm • Confusion, disorientation • Obsessive thoughts • Need for control; feeling out of control • Fear, helplessness, anxiety, anger

In biodynamic sessions, we can sense changes in the system when shock or trauma arises. For example, we can sense when clients are dissociated and not really present in their bodies. At times, we may sense potency being locked up in protective mode, or the subtle motility of the tissues is reduced and the drive or strength of the tide being weak. We can sense and work with activation in the autonomic nervous system, when the sympathetic fight-or-flight system is pulsating wildly through the body, or overwhelm has triggered the parasympathetic system to "play dead." Our work can directly support the nervous system in settling under activated patterns, and can facilitate increased presence in the body where there is a tendency to dissociate. All of this depends on fostering a sense of safety within the practitioner-client relationship.

Safety or Defense: Autonomics in Action

You probably learned something about the autonomic nervous system in biology class in school. Most likely, you were taught about its two parts, the sympathetic, or fight-or-flight system, and the parasympathetic, or rest and rejuvenation system. In life-threatening situations, the parasympathetic system could produce an extreme state of immobility referred to as playing dead or playing possum. Psychotherapists refer to this as a dissociative freeze state. It may also be considered a traumatic shock state. It has commonly been understood that the sympathetic and parasympathetic nervous systems must remain in homeostatic balance in health.

We speed up with sympathetic activation when we run to catch a bus, are under stress, or are being chased by a saber-toothed tiger. Recall that Selye's adaptation response started with alarm, followed by fight-or-flight, and then adaptation. The first two steps involve the sympathetic nervous system. Once we have escaped the tiger, caught the bus, or resolved the stress, we are intended to relax and rejuvenate as our parasympathetic system comes back online. With sympathetic activation, blood is channeled toward the big muscles needed for running or fighting, the muscles of the limbs and jaws. Circulation is reduced for body functions unnecessary for emergencies, such as the digestive and sexual organs. For this reason, people under chronic or severe stress tend to have health problems. Their bodies don't have much chance to regenerate.

We are not intended to stay on sympathetic alert for long. We either outrun the saber-toothed tiger or it catches us in a relatively short time. If we are caught, nature has devised a kind way to protect us from suffering. With a surge of parasympathetic activity, we freeze. The body stops moving, rendering it hopefully less attractive to our predator, who prefers live meat to a possibly diseased, decaying dead carcass. Moreover, we stop feeling. In a dissociated state, if the tiger does decide to go ahead and have us for dinner, we won't feel a thing. We might watch the scene while hovering above the body, but we are spared the pain, as we are no longer connected with our sensations. This is a common experience of trauma survivors, who dissociated from their bodies during the traumatic event and tend to do so again when stressed.

Recall from chapter 2 Porges's discovery of the Polyvagal Theory. Porges recognized that only the old, dorsal vagus nerve is responsible for parasympathetic immobilization. A different, newer, ventral vagus nerve arises from a different brain stem nucleus (nerve center), regulates the heart, supports self-soothing, and is closely associated with other cranial nerves involved with functions essential to social interaction, including facial expressions, speech, hearing, sucking, swallowing, and bonding. He called this the social engagement system and introduced the concept of a triune autonomic nervous system having three components rather than just sympathetic and parasympathetic.[161]

The social engagement nervous system is highly developed in mammals and especially primates, like us humans. Porges recognized that the parasympathetic, sympathetic, and social engagement systems operate as a hierarchy related to their evolutionary development. The parasympathetic system developed first. All creatures have the ability to immobilize when threatened. Even simple unicellular creatures will withdraw in reaction to a toxin or other danger in their environment. The parasympathetic system, present in all vertebrates, specializes in immobilization, both for rest and rejuvenation and for defense.

The sympathetic system evolved later, as creatures developed more ability to mobilize, like amphibians and reptiles with their limbs. When confronted with danger, the sympathetic system enables us to be alert and to fight or fly. When mammals evolved, the third autonomic system came into being as a way to ensure the safety of the young until they are old enough to protect themselves. The social engagement system supports bonding between babies and their mothers (and other caregivers). This involves endearing facial expressions, eye contact, sounds of maternal speech, and baby responses. It underlies breastfeeding, including the sucking and swallowing. This system also facilitates social interactions on all levels. It is the social engagement system that recognizes and fosters safety in our relationships.

Take a moment to think about someone dear to you, someone who, if you saw this person right now, you would both smile and your heart would warm. It could be someone currently

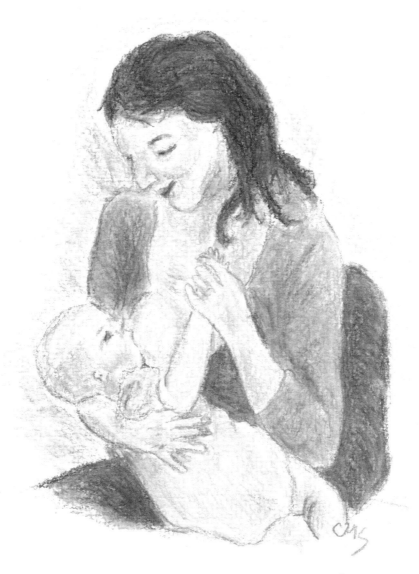

FIGURE 45: Social Engagement Nervous System: Nursing Infant

in your life, but it could also be a person from your past, even a pet you love. What's important is that loving connection between you. Feel your eyes light up when you see them and imagine theirs doing the same. Feel the joy and warmth in your heart at meeting this special person. This is the social engagement system in action! (Thanks to John Chitty for inspiring this exercise.)

Porges noted that, when faced with threat, humans respond first with our most recently evolved system. The social engagement system enables us to look around and read the faces and body expressions of other humans nearby to help us assess if we are in danger. It also supports us in communicating and cooperating with each other to protect ourselves. As individuals, we are easy prey, being relatively small, weak animals. As a group we become a force to contend with. We can build villages, create shelter, share weapons, light fires, and strategize how to protect ourselves in the future.

We are born with our social engagement system online. Even as newborns, we respond to threat with our social engagement system first. If the social nervous system doesn't solve the problem, the sympathetic system takes over. If we are unable to fight or run away, we revert to the oldest, parasympathetic system, withdrawing and freezing, as is common in infants. As described earlier, you can hear this in a baby's cry, beginning as a social calling out for Mother. If Mom doesn't come and the sense of danger persists, the cry begins to sound angry and impatient. These louder cries, as you know if you have ever heard a baby scream, are more difficult to ignore. If they don't bring help, the baby stops crying and becomes very quiet. Such "good babies" who don't fuss are often in a parasympathetic freeze state. These babies haven't simply cried themselves out, as is often believed; they have reached a state of traumatic overwhelm or shock. *Let's take a breath here.* This can be shocking to read!

Consider that little ones are completely dependent on their caregivers for survival. Infants can't mobilize to escape danger. When their attempts at social engagement aren't met, their sympathetic nervous system activates. Their cry becomes louder and more demanding. They are, however, too small and weak to fight off attackers or run from them. Even if there is no aggressor apparent, babies feel unsafe when they are alone because of their extreme dependency and vulnerability. If their sympathetic surge has not brought a rescuing adult to them, they have no way to protect themselves. The only response remaining available to them is to withdraw and freeze. As primates in the jungle, this may be a highly adaptive response for an infant away from its parents. A crying infant attracts danger. A quiet one may be overlooked.

Unfortunately, quiet children are not just overlooked by predators. In modern times, it is not unusual to find children who have been neglected or abused to be in permanent hiding in this subdued parasympathetic state. While some traumatized children seem locked in a sympathetic fight-or-flight rage state and draw the attention of teachers, therapists, and doctors due to their disruptive behavior, others become very quiet. These children often experience further neglect, overlooked by those in charge of them, who assume they are fine because they exhibit no behavior problems. These children, however, are very much in need of help, locked away within a more severe trauma state than their louder peers. (Please note that I am referring here to traumatized children who are withdrawn due to their trauma history. Some children, of course, may be naturally quieter than others by nature. It is important, however, not to assume that a child is quiet because of a natural shyness or introversion in a situation where trauma may be playing a part.) Other traumatized children alternate between aggressive outbursts and quiet withdrawal, as their sympathetic surges burst forth and then their parasympathetic freeze state takes over.

These trauma responses in babies and children are important to understand in biodynamic practice, even when working with adults. As recent research on adverse childhood experiences (ACEs) demonstrates, early trauma often underlies later physical and mental health problems throughout life.[162] Within every adult lives a little one. The quiet, withdrawn child often grows up to be an adult with multiple aches and pains, immune issues, heart and breathing problems, or frequent accidents, possibly due to their inattention to their bodies. They may have difficulty recognizing safety in relationship because they have never experienced it. While they are often shut down emotionally, they may experience high levels of anxiety and fear, interfering with them being able to express their needs or have them met.

Porges points out that our perceptions shift depending on which autonomic nervous system is active.[163] When we are in the defensive sympathetic fight-or-flight or parasympathetic shutdown modes, we tend to sense danger. We are oriented toward threat, on the lookout for where and when it may present next. In this state, a friendly gesture may be misread as an aggressive one, triggering a defensive reaction. This is a common problem with abused children who react violently when another child accidently brushes their arm or reaches out to make friends. Perceiving the friendliness in a friendly gesture requires the social engagement system to be online. In trauma reactions, it tends to go underground, remaining in the background as the sympathetic or parasympathetic systems attempt to deal with potential danger. As Porges notes, this occurs often without awareness, through a process he terms *neuroception*. Different from perception, which involves awareness, neuroception is "detection without awareness."[164] Without the social engagement system acting to inform us, we are unlikely to recognize safety, even when we are safe.

Some of the inspiring value of Porges's theory is the research it has generated in finding ways to stimulate the social engagement system in people with extreme difficulties in social interaction, such as children with autism and other developmental delays.[165] The social engagement system is also helpful in treating trauma as it inhibits, or down regulates, the defensive sympathetic and parasympathetic reactions, enabling traumatized people to recognize when they are safe.

The catch is that the social engagement system comes back online when we feel safe. Neurobiologically speaking, we can either be orienting defensively to avoid danger or we can orient to our social environment. In defensive mode, we notice and react to potentially threatening movements and sounds, scanning our environment for where danger may next present. Ongoing sympathetic activation renders us hypervigilant and unable to rest into social interaction. Parasympathetic dissociative states also interfere with healthy socializing as they lessen our ability to be present and to notice indications of safety or danger. If we dare to enter into relationships when we have dissociative tendencies, we often find ourselves involved with people acting abusively, reminiscent of the situation we are trying to avoid. Our social engagement system, on the other hand, accurately recognizes friendly gestures and detects the human voice within a background of noise. It enables us to know we are not alone and supports human connection.

The question becomes, how do we re-engage the social engagement system when it has been turned off? How do we establish safety for a client who experiences their world as unsafe? Porges has discovered that stimulating the small muscles of the middle ear involved with detecting the higher tones of the human voice can reawaken the social engagement system, producing social behavior in previously isolative autistic children.[166] Similarly, I find that engaging the small muscles of the face and tongue as we do in Continuum can enhance our social orientation. One way we work with the social engagement system in Craniosacral Biodynamics is to ask the client to, as I suggested earlier, recall a loving connection with someone, as the practitioner makes contact with the face or vagus nerve. Another important way is to support the client in orienting to present time and our current relational field, where we can begin to resolve old trauma.

Negotiating Trauma: Coming into Present Time

One of the paradoxical and transformative aspects of implicit traumatic memory is that once it is accessed in a resourced way (through the felt sense), it, by its very nature, changes.

—PETER LEVINE[167]

One of the most helpful ways we can support clients in feeling safe is to be accepting of how they are. Porges points out that evaluative procedures conducted by medical practitioners and therapists immediately provoke a defensive state in clients. He explains:

> I started in my talks to tell clinicians, "Try something different with clients." I said, "Tell your clients who were traumatized that they should celebrate their body's responses, even if the profound physiological and behavioral states that they have experienced currently limit their ability to function in a social world. They should celebrate their body's responses since these responses enable them to survive. It saved their lives. It reduced some of the injury. If they were oppositional during an aggressive traumatic event such as rape, they could have been killed. Tell them to *celebrate* how their body responded instead of making them feel guilty that their body is failing them when they want to be social, and let's see what happens."[168]

In a sense, this attitude of respect and acceptance is characteristic of the biodynamic approach. We are not trying to change anything. We practice orienting to health and how it manifests. For example, Becker noted, "The seeking of health from within is a continuous time, tissue, and tidal effort from conception to the final moments of physiological life. Within every trauma and/or disease entity, there is an effort on the part of body physiology to deliver health mechanisms through the local area of stress to full functioning health capacities."[169]

Where clients are locked in old trauma responses, we can acknowledge this is happening and appreciate the value of these responses in the past and the ongoing expression of health. We can support the client in orienting to present time and the safety that is available now in this relationship. One aspect of this reassurance is our orientation to the health, to what is still working, and the potential available within the wounds. Sometimes, I feel moved to share this verse from Leonard Cohen as a reminder of the potential, or potency, that may be present because of the trauma:

> Ring the bells that still can ring
>
> Forget your perfect offering
>
> There is a crack in everything
>
> That's how the light gets in.
>
> —*"Anthem," Leonard Cohen*

Interestingly, potency may be perceived as light. Remember that Sutherland referred to it as "liquid light."

Within a biodynamic context, we talk with our clients to support them in being present and not overwhelmed when old trauma stored in their body arises. It can be helpful to reassure the client that the trembling occurring is not a bad thing, that it is the energy of the old trauma releasing. We can reassure them that we understand and are comfortable holding their process. Often clients feel that their history or their emotions are too much. They are too much for them and certainly too much for another person to witness or hold. Knowing that the practitioner has the ability and willingness to be with what arises, and can support them in being able to be with it, can be very soothing.

For practitioners to be able to hold trauma arising in clients requires that we do our own work. Trainees are expected to receive ongoing, regular sessions themselves to help them address aspects of their own history arising as their own armor melts. This enables them to be more present and perceptive with their clients. Ongoing supervision is also important for practitioners as support in working with their own history when it is touched by their clients' process. Psychotherapy is also useful at times as support in being able to be with this territory.

In Craniosacral Biodynamics, we understand that potency coalesces to protect when trauma occurs, and that this protective function of potency can shift to a healing function when the person feels safe enough to settle within the relational field. Potency will choose an inertial fulcrum to work with. When supported within a safe relational field in an adequately resourced state, the forces held within the tissues will be discharged. We sense softening, enlivening, and increased coherence as the trauma resolves. Through this process, we often encounter emotional or psychological correlates. If the fulcrum arose through injury, the event responsible may have included intense fear, which the client may feel during the healing process. Usually, the autonomic nervous system is involved. There may be a sudden increase in heart rate, the skin reddens, the person feels hot, or they may feel like jumping off the table and running out of the room. They may feel angry, impatient, or restless. It can be helpful to acknowledge these feelings, and that may have been how the person felt at the time of the trauma.

Sometimes it is helpful to simply explain how the nervous system works with trauma. It can be important to understand that we are designed to shake off our sympathetic energy once the stress is over. If we remain frozen or we are stopped from releasing the held energy by cultural expectations, well-meaning others, or medications, the fight-or-flight impulses remain trapped in our nervous system, waiting for an opportunity to be expressed. The trembling or anger or feeling of wanting to run away can be indications of this energy. Simply acknowledging and accepting the reaction may enable it to soften. When challenging feelings arise, it is usually helpful to find a way to support the client in being with them. This is about being able to be present with them, rather than falling into and drowning in what trauma therapist Peter Levine has termed the "trauma vortex."[170]

Levine has revolutionized trauma therapies in recent years. The Somatic Experiencing work he has developed is very complementary to the biodynamic approach. Trauma work in Craniosacral Biodynamics was originally influenced by Core Process Psychotherapy (CPP), mentioned earlier as an influence Sills brought into the work. Founded in the 1980s by Maura Sills, assisted by Franklyn Sills, CPP incorporates Buddhist principles into psychotherapy, supporting clients in learning to be present with their process through mindful, present-time-oriented awareness. I have heard Franklyn Sills speak about his first time meeting Peter Levine. Both were presenting at a conference. After hearing each other speak, they agreed that their approaches to trauma were similar. After this, Sills began incorporating Levine's terminology into the biodynamic training.

As part of our work with trauma, we consider our ability to process information when resourced or traumatized. In our usual resilient state, we can easily shift between what is called bottom-up and top-down processing. "Bottom-up" refers to the stream of sensory information traveling from our senses into our brain, where it can be assessed and responded to appropriately. "Top-down" refers to the brainy part of the communication, where cortical parts of our brain evaluate and moderate our sensory input from all over the body and respond accordingly.

With unresolved trauma, the easy shifting between these two modes of processing is interrupted. We may become locked in survival mode, with our top-down processing largely lost. Instead of thinking through and integrating incoming stimuli, we often react from within a cycling stress response. All stimuli become additional stress. Our cortex is less available to think things through; we tend to be run by survival emotions, like anger and fear, and the hypervigilance associated with them. The neural pathways involved become overstimulated and oversensitized.

Supporting our clients in orienting to present time and the safety of the current relational field helps to reawaken the social engagement system and related cortical structures capable of modulating the stress response. We can also support the system as a whole in orienting to the resource of stillness and the deeper tides, enhancing the ability to settle under the activation. Orienting to sensation within our verbal, relational field supports integration, where the top-down and bottom-up processing can begin to be more fluid again. We also can work specifically to support normalizing overactive, sensitized nerves, so they can return to the original blueprint for their function.

Revisiting Resource

An essential aspect of our approach to trauma is to stay resourced in present time. Resource, as discussed in chapter 3, refers to what supports us in the midst of whatever our experience is. We generally begin biodynamic sessions by helping our clients orient to resource. This becomes the starting point and foundation for our work together. We may ask for a word or phrase that we can use during the session to remind the client of resource should this seem useful. Then, if trauma arises, or if the client begins to demonstrate some autonomic activation, we can help them reorient to resource. This supports them in being able to stay present, to witness the trauma reaction or memory, without getting lost in it.

Sometimes clients misunderstand or mistrust this approach. They believe, as did therapists for many years, that healing trauma requires recalling every detail of the story and cathartically expressing the emotions associated with the event. They fear that orienting to resource when trauma memories arise will suppress the memories and interfere with trauma resolution. Trauma research, however, demonstrates the opposite. Cathartic techniques and retelling the story of the traumatic event may increase awareness of what happened, but tend to reinforce the neurological pathways associated with trauma responses, causing them to persist. Revisiting the trauma in a slower, more regulated way, supported by awareness of resource and present-time support, enables the nervous system to release its trauma-related charge in a manageable way. The memories can be integrated. New neural pathways involving speech and the social nervous system can be established as the trauma history is met in a way that is not overwhelming or retraumatizing.

Simple questions we ask when trauma arises are, "How is that for you?" "How is it for you to be with this?" or "Do you feel like you can be with this?" We usually remind the person of the resources we talked about at the beginning of the session. If we have helped them to have a felt sense of the resource in the body, it can be easier to access this sense again when reminded. Other simple questions to help the client be present might be, "Can you feel my hand making contact with your shoulder (or wherever the contact is)? How is that for you?" In biodynamic training, we incorporate these kinds of verbal skills to use when working with clients during sessions.

In biodynamic session work, we support clients in practicing mindful awareness. This becomes a useful resource if trauma presents. Mindfulness involves observing what arises, including body sensations, thoughts, feelings, and emotions. We ask our clients from time to time what they are experiencing, and support them in reporting in a body-centered way, referring to sensations as much as possible. For example, if I ask you what you are feeling, you might tell me that you feel OK (a common nonspecific response!). I might ask you, "What in your body tells you that you are OK?" or "Where do you sense that in your body?" Then, you begin to notice a sense of relaxation and softness, or a comfortable warmth, or how your body is resting into the treatment table. This is a simple mindfulness practice. *You might take a moment to practice this right now, just checking in again with what you are aware of in your breath and body.*

Mindfulness has been shown to rewire the brain in ways that support us in being in present time, rather than being lost in trauma memories.[171] In traumatized individuals, parts of the brain associated with sympathetic arousal and alertness to danger tend to be overactive. The amygdala, for example, as mentioned earlier functions like a sentry in the brain, always scanning incoming sensory input and comparing it with memories of the past for indications of danger. This is important but, if it is overly active, it keeps the sympathetic nervous system stimulated and the person can't relax. The social engagement system remains behind the scenes as orientation to potential threat persists, based on past experience. The individual isn't really in the present.

Practicing mindfulness activates a different part of the brain, the prefrontal cortex, which relates to awareness of present time. It is closely associated with the social engagement system, and can support us in coming into relationship with those we are actually currently present with. As the client comes into relationship with the practitioner, they can begin to sense safety where they may have been previously lost in repeated reruns of a less-safe past. The body can then begin to let go and release its hold on the past. Trauma can begin to resolve. The potential it obscured is free to express. Life can begin again.

8
Next Steps

In this chapter, I would like to invite you to review your experience of reading this book and note for yourself: *What has touched you in this process? Are you changed in any way through reading these pages? Are you inspired? Are you left with curiosity, questions, or an impulse to explore this biodynamic territory further?* This chapter discusses options for further study and discovery. These range from finding a biodynamic practitioner and receiving the work yourself, to taking an introductory seminar or committing to the full two-year practitioner training. Potential directions for postgraduate studies are also covered here, as are complementary or preparatory studies or therapies that can support you in deepening into Craniosacral Biodynamics both as a practitioner and a client.

The first section discusses major paradigm shifts in perception and being that usually accompany a biodynamic journey, as well as emphases in the training curriculum. This is likely to be of interest even if you are intending to receive the work without studying it yourself. The second section is about finding a biodynamic practitioner who is right for you and discusses receiving the work. In that a significant aspect of becoming a practitioner is to receive biodynamic work, this section will be useful for prospective trainees as well as those solely interested in receiving work. The third section describes the curriculum of the practitioner training as it is taught and has developed at the Karuna Institute, including some of the rationale behind the curriculum design. This section includes prerequisites and guidance in preparing to begin the training. This will be primarily of interest to those planning to take the training to become a practitioner or to deepen their Craniosacral Therapy skills. Details may vary for trainings outside of Karuna, but this section can give you at least a general idea of how the foundation trainings work. Postgraduate options are discussed in the fourth section, directed at those who have already completed a biodynamic training or who like to plan further ahead. Finally, the concluding chapter covers helpful resources for learning more, including books, videos, and websites specifically on Craniosacral Biodynamics, as well as on trauma, prenatal and birth issues, and anatomy and physiology.

A Biodynamic Journey: Paradigm Shifts and Transformation

A biodynamic journey, whether as client or developing practitioner, inevitably involves dramatic shifts in perception and ways of viewing your world. These shifts accompany changes in your paradigm for life, health, and being. While transformation at this level can be disorienting, it can also provide powerful rewards, enabling you to embrace your body, life, and relationships in ways you never have before.

A first paradigm shift for many entering the biodynamic training or receiving sessions involves our relationship to health and disease. Craniosacral Biodynamics is founded on a basic principle of Osteopathy, from which it has emerged. We orient to inherent health, rather than to disease, problems, issues, and how to fix them. This is a major shift in perspective for most clients and students of Craniosacral Biodynamics. In our modern Western culture, health is valued but poorly understood and rarely focused on. When we go to a doctor or health practitioner, of course our intention is to improve our health, but our focus is on what is keeping us from experiencing health. We complain about our back pain, headaches, anxiety, insomnia, lack of concentration, arthritis, fatigue, allergies, etc. When I ask clients about what they are experiencing or aware of in their bodies, their first response is almost always about their discomfort. After hearing about all their aches and pains, I also often ask, what feels OK in your body just now? I have seen clients experience a major life shift because of this question. It may have never occurred to them to consider something feeling OK. We are taught from the time we are little to only reference our bodies if they are problematic. How often do you ask someone "How are you?" and receive an exact reply describing all the good feelings and experiences the person is having? How often do you note these expressions of health in your own body?

This brings us to another area of potential change for people on their biodynamic journeys. Biodynamic Craniosacral Therapy includes a mindful approach to our experience. This involves developing awareness of our current physical sensations, as well as our thoughts, emotions, and feelings. Although mindfulness is growing in popularity, this kind of awareness is again counter to our modern Western paradigm. You probably learned about René Descartes, the father of modern philosophy, in school. Descartes was the seventeenth-century French philosopher often considered responsible for the mind-body split so epidemic in our modern world: "I think therefore I am." With this declaration, which apparently emerged from his doubting his own sensations, Descartes established the thinking mind as all-important.

Rational thinking is of course important, but Craniosacral Biodynamics involves enhancing awareness of physical sensations as a way to support presence and trauma resolution, both aspects of health. For those of us raised to ignore or cut ourselves off from our bodily sensations, returning to them can literally be mind-blowing. We may discover how inaccurate our beliefs and assumptions can be! For most of us, splitting off our awareness from our bodies has been associated with intolerable experiences when we were little.[172] Whether we consider these experiences to be traumatic or simply part of becoming socialized, we have learned to listen to our thoughts while dismissing the somatosensory information, which informs them.[173] When we are guided to reorient to our sensations, we can begin to perceive differently, often freshly.

Through receiving biodynamic sessions, we not only tend to become more aware of the body, but we also may begin to have more pleasant sensations. As the nervous system settles, and we drop under our usual tendencies, we may have a sense of the body melting, tissues shifting as old patterns dissolve and become less important. This can lead to shifts in our perceptions and view of the world. For example chronic pain is often accompanied by depression, where our worldview becomes more negative, hopeless, and narrow. As tissues shift and pain lessens, the depression may begin to lift. It can be like starting life again.

The most dramatic experience I witnessed of this phenomenon was with an elderly woman brought to me by her daughter for treatment. She was suffering intensely from the unrelenting pain of fibromyalgia. Her life had essentially stopped. She felt hopeless, shut down, and suicidal. I was amazed when, after just two sessions, her daughter reported that her mother was back to her bridge games and enjoying life again! She continued to receive sessions to support further healing, but her outlook had completely changed.

We don't need to be depressed and suicidal to experience shifts in mindset or perception through Craniosacral Biodynamics. Most people find their outlook changes at least in some ways during a course of treatment.

One common kind of shift is that people receiving biodynamic sessions usually find themselves becoming calmer and more relaxed. A major effect of Craniosacral

Biodynamics is slowing down and settling nervous system activation. This can feel wonderfully relaxing, but it may also take some adjusting to. In our fast-paced modern world, we may feel at a disadvantage being slowed down. We may feel vulnerable. This often reflects our history more than our current reality. We may have learned to speed up and stay task-oriented as a way to protect ourselves, or to get the recognition, appreciation, and love we needed back then. Slowing down may bring us face-to-face with long-forgotten or buried feelings of unworthiness, fear, shame, rejection, anger at how we have been mistreated, or the exhaustion of protecting ourselves for years. As our nervous system settles, it can shift from focusing on danger, threat, and defense to our more essential nature, characterized by warmth, presence, open-heartedness, and even love. We may undergo a shift of identity.

Who are we, if not our defensive personality structure we have always known? As the defensive patterning in the nervous system shifts, we begin to access a different system of processing experience, the social engagement nervous system. As our neurobiology shifts, we are not only calmer and more present, but also more accurately able to perceive the people who are actually with us now rather than seeing them as representatives or reminders of those we found hurtful or dangerous in the past. We return to our intrinsic friendliness, playfulness, and natural social intelligence. In the process, old unresolved traumas and issues may come to the surface, ready for healing. Your biodynamic practitioner is trained to support you in being able to be present with what arises, without getting lost in it or retraumatizing yourself. In this vein, you may learn some valuable methods for staying present, such as some of the grounding and resourcing practices presented earlier in this book.

Many unexpected changes can occur for biodynamic clients and students. It is not unusual to start seeing colors more brightly, thinking more clearly, having more energy, resting more deeply, and experiencing more order and creativity. I have had clients go home and suddenly feel compelled to organize their living space. You may feel like you want to go for a walk, start an exercise program, or eat more healthily. As your system orients more to its inherent health, it becomes easier to choose health-supporting options.

As your body and heart open in this work, it is not uncommon for your relationships to shift. Abusive behavior becomes less tolerable. You may find yourself being more articulate and assertive in relation to your needs. You also may have more compassion for your partner, friends, or others, feeling more patient or understanding than you have in the past. I can almost guarantee that, as you deepen in this biodynamic journey, change will happen.

We will discuss more thoroughly some of the paradigm and perceptual shifts involved in learning and practicing Craniosacral Biodynamics in a later section. First, let's look at how to start receiving sessions, if you are not already.

Receiving Biodynamic Sessions: Finding a Practitioner and Discovering More of Yourself

Receiving biodynamic sessions supports personal healing and is also an important way to begin learning the work if you are interested in becoming a practitioner. We generally require applicants for the practitioner training to receive sessions before beginning the training as a way to understand more clearly what they are moving into. Taking the training also involves exchanging practice sessions during class, as well as receiving sessions from a graduate between modules. The training requirement is generally to receive at least ten sessions from a professional who has studied this type of Craniosacral Biodynamics. This is to support your own healing, as well as learning more about the work directly through your own body and healing. Ten sessions over two years, however, is extremely minimal. We usually recommend receiving biodynamic sessions on a weekly or biweekly basis to support ongoing healing and change. When working with clients, I usually recommend weekly sessions if possible for a period of time, depending on the nature and severity of the client's condition. Once a foundation has been established and the person experiences relative health, frequency of sessions can be reduced as needed.

Some clients love the work and its effects so much that they want to keep coming every week. There is no detriment to receiving this work frequently. Craniosacral Biodynamics is not about applying techniques to create change in your body or interfere with how it is already coping with whatever it needs to handle. Craniosacral Biodynamics is much more about supporting your system to settle under its activations and historical patterns, and to connect more fully with the intrinsic health always present within you. While change often results from this shift in orientation, it generally occurs gently in ways you can readily integrate.

Having said this, clients often seek Craniosacral Biodynamics because they have specific issues. They may come with headaches, anxiety, back or joint pain, or other chronic pain issues. They may have chronic neurological conditions like multiple sclerosis, or they may have had a stroke or brain injury. They often seek help for post-traumatic stress disorder or other effects of trauma from their past, including prenatal and birth trauma. Some have insomnia or learning problems, or children may come because of behavior problems. Some clients simply know they are too stressed in their lives and come to relax. Craniosacral Biodynamics can be helpful with any of these kinds of issues because it helps your system to find its health, resetting your nervous system and releasing the forces of old traumas, injuries, etc., still active in your body.

I suggest that in seeking a practitioner you begin with clarifying your own intention in receiving the work. Are you just curious? Do you have a specific health problem you want addressed? Is there something in your personal history that is nagging you and wanting attention? Are you hoping to find a new way to relieve stress or enhance your general state of well-being? It can be useful to take some time to sit with this question and perhaps write a paragraph or at least a sentence as a statement about what you are looking for. Once you have clarified this, your intention can guide you in knowing what to ask your potential practitioner, to help ensure you find someone who is a good match for what you want and need.

Choosing a Practitioner: Beginning a Therapeutic Relationship

Biodynamic sessions also can be helpful because of the relationship you develop with your practitioner. As described earlier in this book, the "relational field" is an important aspect of this work. Practitioners are trained to support their clients in feeling safe and settled in their presence. It is important in receiving this work that you feel comfortable with your practitioner. I recommend talking with prospective practitioners before having your first session to get a sense of how you feel with them. Do you feel at ease? Do you have a sense of wanting to be around this person more? Does your body relax at all when you are talking with them? Do you feel comfortable to tell them about your issues and intentions? Or do you find your body tensing as you interact? Do you feel panicky, ill at ease, or mistrusting? While you may recognize such feelings as your typical response to the potential for interpersonal closeness, it is important to consider your feelings and sensations in deciding whom to work with.

These responses are most readily sensed in face-to-face contact with another person. In these days of digital online communications, it is not unusual for clients to make appointments by email or even via an online calendar on the practitioner's website. There is, however, usually an option to call the practitioner or arrange to talk with them briefly by phone. (If this is not presented as an option, you might request it.) Even though it takes more time to talk rather than sending a quick email,

I recommend giving yourself a chance to at least hear the practitioner's voice before making your appointment. This gives you important information and may also help you to be able to settle and receive more easily in the first session.

We are designed to assess strangers through our visual and auditory senses. This is elucidated by Stephen Porges, whose polyvagal nervous system theory and concept of the social engagement nervous system mentioned earlier have changed the face of therapy in recent years. Porges emphasizes the importance of "prosody" or tone of voice for supporting us in shifting from defensive nervous system stances to a more socially engaged state, where we can perceive the safety available in the current relationship.[174] Hearing your practitioner's voice can let you know you feel safe and can relax in their presence. Seeing the practitioner's face can also give you valuable information, but this is not always essential once you have heard their voice. These days, you can also check out potential practitioners by watching videos they have posted online. As you watch, observe your own reaction, how relaxed you feel, and your sense of wanting to be with this person or not. Trust what you sense!

Having said this, who you choose as your practitioner may depend solely on where you live. Craniosacral Biodynamics, also referred to as Biodynamic Craniosacral Therapy or BCST, is still a relatively new field that is gradually becoming better known. There may not be a large variety of practitioners available to you locally. To assist you in your search, here are some tips.

Questions to Ask a Potential Practitioner

If you are hoping to work with a biodynamically oriented craniosacral therapist, your most important questions will relate to your potential practitioner's training. You can ask them about what kind of Craniosacral Therapy they practice, where and with whom they trained, what a session looks like, what is their orientation in Craniosacral work. It is also important to find out logistical details, like location, length of sessions, fees charged, cancellation policy, etc. If you have a specific issue you want addressed, you may want to ask what kind of experience your practitioner has with that particular problem. While a practitioner may be a good match for you even if they haven't worked with your issue before, how they respond to your question can give you information about how they work and how they will be with you. It can be helpful to talk with the practitioner enough to give yourself a sense of how comfortable you feel with them. Since this work depends on the relational field being able to settle, does this feel like someone you can trust and settle with? You may not have logical reasons for being drawn to the practitioner; you may just have an intuitive sense that this is or isn't the one for you, or that this person has something to offer you at this time.

If you are interested in training to become a practitioner, it is useful to receive sessions from someone who has trained at the school you are planning to attend. This will give you a sense of how you might practice after the training and what the training will provide you with. It can be informative to receive from different practitioners if you are planning to take the training, as you learn from each one. Each practitioner has their own style and approach, informed not only by their training, but also by their personality and other clinical and life experience. I encourage you, as a potential trainee, to ask questions. Be curious about what your practitioner is doing (or not doing) and why. Not all practitioners will be comfortable or articulate talking about what they do, but you can learn from those who are. Listen for what resonates with you. What attracts you? What inspires you?

Where to Find a Practitioner

Finding a biodynamic practitioner isn't always as easy as we might hope. In North America, biodynamic therapists register with the Biodynamic Craniosacral Therapy Association of North America (BCTA/NA). The association website, www.craniosacraltherapy .org, provides a listing of practitioners by state or province. These practitioners have all graduated from a training with a BCTA/NA-approved teacher, following the training guidelines as listed on the website. Some postgraduate training or supervision is required to renew registration each year. The association does not however regulate the specifics taught in the curriculum. Practitioners listed have a wide variety of training and approaches, even while all use the term *biodynamic*. Furthermore, not all biodynamic practitioners in America are registered with the BCTA/NA. Some schools have a listing of their own graduates. While these will help you determine if a person has graduated from a particular school, the list of graduates doesn't indicate if the graduate has ongoing supervision or postgraduate training. Some schools list advanced practitioners, usually indicating those listed have engaged in a certain amount of postgraduate work.

Finding a Biodynamic Craniosacral Therapist in Your Area

On a practical level, there are several ways to find a biodynamic practitioner in your area. One is to contact biodynamic schools. Karuna Institute, for example, can offer you a list of therapists trained at Karuna who practice near you. There are also associations in different parts of the world involved in registering practitioners. I am most familiar with the BCTA/NA, which registers practitioners primarily in the US and Canada. It also registers teachers, through whom you can also find practitioners in your area. On the BCTA/NA website, www.craniosacraltherapy.org, you can find practitioners and teachers in different regions. Registered practitioners use "RCST"" (Registered Craniosacral Therapist) after their name. These practitioners have not only graduated from an approved training, or the equivalent, but have also maintained required supervision/continuing education requirements and ethical standards. This is also true of the Craniosacral Therapy Association (CSTA) of the UK, which maintains its own list of registered practitioners at www.craniosacral.co.uk. Note that the CSTA is not limited to biodynamic practitioners, so you will want to find out about a practitioner's training background. Other countries have similar associations and can help you find registered practitioners. There are also biodynamic practitioners across Europe and in South Africa, Australia, New Zealand, Israel, India, and other countries at the time of this writing. The work seems to be spreading throughout the world, so if you live somewhere not listed here, have hope and do some research. You may discover you live next door to a wonderful biodynamic practitioner! A list of associations is included in Chapter Nine on Resources for Learning More.

A worldwide association, International Affiliation of Biodynamic Trainings (IABT), originally designed to support and link biodynamic schools around the world, provides lists of graduates of these schools on its website at http://biodynamic-craniosacral.org or www.iabt.org. Consider that graduates are people who have completed the training program, which is different from being registered and maintaining requirements for registration. These usually include ethical standards, as well as supervision and postgraduate education. In contrast to registration with a professional association, like BCTA/NA, BCST designation given to graduates by IABT schools is comparable to an academic degree earned by completing a university program. For example, I completed a master's degree in dance/movement therapy. In order to work as a dance/movement therapist, however, I needed to then register with the American Dance Therapy Association. This required many hours of practice with supervision and other postgraduate activities. I have since dropped that registration and no longer officially practice dance/movement therapy. I will always, however, have my degree in the field, whether I practice or not. In other words, seeing that someone has graduated from a training program does not give you information about current practice. It simply indicates they have completed this training.

Some IABT schools offer an "Advanced Biodynamic Practitioner" (ABP), somewhat comparable to professional registration, since the "Advanced Biodynamic Diploma"

(ABD) requires further postgraduate studies. Professional registration, however, generally requires ongoing continuing education and supervision, intended to ensure standards of practice are maintained. Again, having taken advanced courses in dance/movement therapy wouldn't necessarily ensure that I was professionally registered or practicing as a dance/movement therapist.

If you feel drawn to a practitioner, particularly one who is not registered with an association, I again recommend arranging to talk with them before your first session to determine what they practice and if you feel drawn or comfortable to work with them. It may not be important to you whether they are registered or not. It will undoubtedly be important that you feel at ease with them.

If you choose to find a practitioner from a particular school, you can find biodynamic schools listed at the IABT website (http://biodynamic-craniosacral.org or www.iabt.org). These include schools around the world.

Confusion in the Field

It is easy to become confused as you seek a biodynamic practitioner because the use of the term *biodynamic* has become widespread and does not necessarily relate to the particular form of work discussed in this book. For example, I have been assured by some biodynamic cranial osteopaths that they often work somewhat differently from how we do, although there are overlaps in our work. There are also other craniosacral therapists who use the term *biodynamic,* derived from different sources, who also practice differently. Adding to the confusion, other kinds of bodywork and psychotherapy also use the term and may differ considerably from Biodynamic Craniosacral Therapy.

Please note that I use the word *different* for the sake of clarity, not judgment. It is not that one type of work is better or more effective than another. Because there are several forms of work using the same or similar terms, however, it can be difficult to determine just from the name what kind of work is actually being offered. If you want to experience or learn more about what is described in this book, my intention is to help you find practitioners doing this type of work!

If you are unsure, I recommend checking to see if the practitioner you have found is registered. It is possible that, if they are not registered, they are nonetheless practicing in this way. Also, some who are registered may be practicing differently. You may then want to interview them to get a sense of how they work and how you feel with them.

In seeking a practitioner, it can be helpful to know more about their background, where they have trained and what their training entailed. Many biodynamic practitioners have training in other modalities, which may influence how they work. For example, they may incorporate their knowledge of homeopathy or trauma therapy into their biodynamic session work. Most biodynamic trainings require that their trainees have at least some experience as some kind of health or healing practitioner before taking the training. The next section will help you understand more about how biodynamic practitioners are trained, particularly at Karuna Institute and other foundation trainings taught by Franklyn Sills and staff outside of Karuna.

Becoming a Practitioner of Craniosacral Biodynamics

Are you considering becoming a practitioner of Craniosacral Biodynamics? You may have read this book because you already intended to become a practitioner. Or perhaps you feel inspired to take the training after reading the book. (I'd love to hear from you if that is the case!) Or you may already be a practitioner interested in deepening your skills. A section in the next chapter discusses postgraduate training for those who are already biodynamic practitioners. If you currently practice Craniosacral Therapy, but have not studied a biodynamic approach, my intention here is to provide an overview of the practitioner training, which may be of interest to you. We often have experienced cranial osteopaths, as well as craniosacral therapists with different approaches, attend our trainings. This following also offers guidance in choosing the training that is right for you, and some other important factors to consider in embarking on the biodynamic journey. You may also find this section informative if you are receiving biodynamic sessions and want to learn more or to understand more of your practitioner's background and perspective.

Overview of the Foundation Training in Craniosacral Biodynamics

The biodynamic training is generally at least two years long, the equivalent of about fifty days. Usually, this is offered as ten five-day modules, although variations have been developed to help make the training more affordable and easier to access in terms of the number of days or trips required to participate. In North America, biodynamic trainings are regulated by the Biodynamic Craniosacral Therapy Association of North America (BCTA/NA). Teachers in America are approved and certified by the BCTA/NA and may conduct their own trainings. The BCTA/NA website, www.craniosacraltherapy.org, includes guidelines that trainings are required to meet if their graduates are to be eligible for registration with the association. In Europe and the UK, schools, rather than teachers, are approved. Graduates of these schools are assumed to have met basic requirements to be eligible for registration where local registration bodies exist. For more information on Biodynamic and Craniosacral Therapy organizations, please refer to the section "Where to Find a Practitioner," in this chapter, and listings in the next chapter.

The model informing this book is based on the program offered and developed at Karuna Institute in England. Franklyn Sills has developed the curriculum there over many years, supported by a dedicated team of tutors. Most of the teachers of Craniosacral Biodynamics around the world outside of the field of Osteopathy have either studied with Sills or with someone who studied with him. In that the training has shifted dramatically over the years, however, what is actually being taught in various trainings varies greatly. Therefore, I recommend doing some research of your own before enrolling in a training to make sure it is a good fit for you. Again, I suggest reviewing what has touched you most deeply from this book, what resonates with you most strongly, and then interviewing your potential teachers or schools to check that those aspects will be addressed. You may, of course, find aspects of other trainings that you are interested in that are different from what we offer at Karuna. I feel it is important that you investigate what is being offered by any given training so you can make an informed choice. Two years and ten modules is a major commitment in terms of time, money, and energy. It is worth your while to ensure before you begin that the training you choose is the right one for you.

Most trainings offer a short, two- to five-day introductory seminar to give you a sense of what the training is about and to make sure it is what you want. Again, two years is a big commitment! If you decide to take the training, I can almost guarantee you will go through profound changes within yourself, your life, and your relationships. I have never experienced a biodynamic training where trainees don't at some point find they are seeing themselves and others, and even the world, differently. Let's look at what is involved in the training curriculum that might contribute to such shifts.

Perceptual Shifts

I have heard it said that biodynamic practitioner training is a program in perception. A major intention of the training is to deepen under our everyday perceptions of form and structure to enhance perception of the forces responsible for that structure. As described in an earlier chapter, these include both universal biodynamic forces and conditional forces. Biodynamic forces are manifestations of the mysterious source we call the Breath of Life. A major aspect of the training is about learning to perceive and support the subtle rhythmic manifestations of the Breath of Life that we call Primary Respiration and the deeper ground of dynamic stillness. We also learn to recognize manifestations of conditional forces. These are often sensed as faster, more variable, less coherent rhythms we call the cranial rhythmic impulse (CRI), as well as areas of inertia, density, and patterning within the tissues.

The essence of the biodynamic approach is of shifting our orientation from these superficial tissue expressions to the deeper forces organizing them. This is a perceptual shift, relating to the paradigm shifts in the biodynamic journey described earlier in this chapter. Shifting perception is demonstrated by the Gestalt images you may have encountered that appear as two completely different pictures depending on where or how you focus. The most famous of these figure-ground drawings is probably the faces-vase drawing in figure 46.

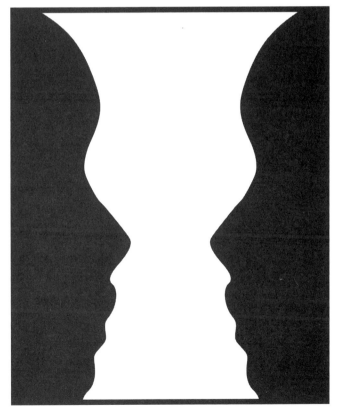

FIGURE 46: Figure Ground: Faces and Vase
Source: https://en.wikipedia.org/wiki/Figure–ground_%28perception%29#/media/File:
Cup_or_faces_paradox.svg. Accessed June 21, 2015.

What do you see when you look at this image? You are likely to either see the white vase in the center or the two black profiles on the sides. In Craniosacral Biodynamics, we practice widening our field of perception in order to view more of the whole. How much of the whole of this image are you able to perceive? Once you are able to see both images separately, your perception may alternate between the two. It may take awhile for you to be able to take in the whole scene.

Our perception in Craniosacral Biodynamics develops in a similar way. Usually, trainees arrive with some awareness of what we might call the figure: the tissues and structures presenting in the body. When we first make contact with a client's body, we might sense how hard or soft the tissues under our hands are. We may feel rapid pulsations relating to the activated sympathetic nervous system common to most people living in our overstimulating, accelerated twenty-first century. Or we may sense a dissociative deadness. The tissues seem uninhabited, as if no one is home. We may sense the tissues being pulled in one direction or another as chronic patterns present themselves. In Craniosacral Biodynamics, this is a starting point. We settle ourselves as practitioners, support the client in settling under all of this CRI activation, and wait for the deeper forces and the inherent treatment plan to arise. This requires a deepening and widening of our own perception.

As mentioned earlier, most biodynamic trainings have as a prerequisite that potential trainees are already practitioners of some kind. Many are massage therapists, acupuncturists, physio- or occupational therapists, nurses, doctors, osteopaths, homeopaths, naturopaths, or bodyworkers of some kind. While some arrive with a background in other kinds of therapeutic practice, often psychotherapy or counseling, most have at least some training in making physical contact and sensing the physical body in some way. Often they arrive with years of training and experience in their field of expertise. They are accustomed to focusing on the symptoms or complaints their clients present and have a toolbox full of techniques to help resolve these problems. It is sometimes a relief but usually also a challenge to let go of their familiar mode of perception, involving analysis of presenting issues and application of techniques to fix them.

Learning a biodynamic mode of perception involves shifting focus from this presenting figure to a wider orientation to more of the background, including the underlying forces. It also involves learning to sit back and allow the body to work, rather than actively doing or applying techniques. This is not only a shift in perception, but also in being. Trainees tend to undergo major changes in how they interact with their lives as they learn to relinquish active doing modes and relax into more of a being state.

These shifts can be challenging as well as profoundly rewarding. One factor contributing to the challenge is that Craniosacral Biodynamics involves learning to function in ways unfamiliar to our modern Western culture. We learn in school to narrow our focus and "pay attention." Our subtle perceptual abilities, natural in small children, are socialized out of us, usually by the time we start school. Modern Western culture focuses on the concrete. Our science has rejected any evidence that cannot be easily measured, replicated, or recorded. While quantum physics is starting to influence the modern world to include more subtle realms in our view of reality, most of us have not been raised to honor our most subtle perceptions.

Learning Craniosacral Biodynamics involves learning to trust at a deep level. We must learn to trust our subtle perceptions, what we know within, and that something unfamiliar or unknown may have value. During the training, students practice their skills with each other and are encouraged to exchange feedback regarding what they are sensing. If I am sensing a subtle rhythm, I might be more inclined to trust that perception if my practice client describes sensing something similar. Trainees are also required to give a minimum of 150 practice sessions with nonpaying clients outside of class, with supervision from the training tutors. Practice clients are given a form to sign giving their consent to be practice clients, rather than actual clients, understanding that these sessions are intended for the trainee's learning. While the practice client usually benefits from the sessions, the trainee has certain skills and holds to practice and needs to feel free to experiment. It is important to have these sessions as an opportunity to not be the all-knowing expert professional, but to be able to learn from mistakes, to get feedback from the practice client, and to try out new skills. Again, this can be challenging for trainees who often already have a busy practice and are accustomed to being paid for their expertise.

One of the greatest challenges of the biodynamic training can be returning to what is called in Buddhism "beginners' mind." While the training includes learning relevant anatomy, physiology, and neurobiology, it is important to be able to follow Sutherland's advice from many years ago to know what we need to know, but then put it "behind the curtain."[175] As Sills elucidates:

> You need all you know, all of your understanding and skills, yet you need to allow it all to go behind the curtain, to become unseen. You must enter that SeaAroundUs naked of the need to change anything, to analyze or diagnose anything, totally open to the present moment, listening for the healing intentions of the Breath of Life.[176]

The paradigm shift involved in learning to be and perceive in this sacred way is a major reason the training is spread out over at least two years. While it was initially a one-year training, Sills realized this was not long enough for students to deepen into the perceptual fields of truly biodynamic work. As mentioned in chapter 1 on the history of Craniosacral Biodynamics, the curriculum has evolved over many years and dramatically shifted around 2002 to 2006, as Sills and the tutor team at Karuna realized they were not teaching what they were practicing. Sills had initially designed the curriculum based on the traditional osteopathic training he had experienced, beginning with more biomechanical skills. He later realized these are not really relevant to a biodynamic approach and may even interfere with developing biodynamic perceptual skills.

While many osteopathic trainings don't include biodynamic skills, those that do usually emphasize more biomechanical practices first. They follow the perceptual journey originally taken by Sutherland as his cranial skills developed, beginning with cranial bone motion, then including soft tissues, fluids, and eventually the underlying energetic forces organizing them. The latter relate to the final decade of Sutherland's life, when his orientation became less biomechanical.

Sills had believed it was important to include the more biomechanical skills in the training, but gradually realized that perceiving and working with deeper forces did not require extensive work with the tissues and fluids they organize. He noted that having established more biomechanical skills could actually impede the subtler biodynamic perception. Working on a biomechanical level demands very specific knowledge and skill in assessing and altering tissue patterns. A biodynamic approach, however, requires letting go of any need to know every detail and control these patterns, enabling us to settle under these superficial expressions of deeper forces organizing them and allowing the profound "Intelligence with a capital I" to do its work.

Relinquishing control in this way again requires trust. It also challenges us to let go of our ego's needs to control, to know, to be the expert, or to rescue, fix, or be successful. Over time, we learn that the Intelligence of the potency (embodied life force within the fluids) is far more capable than we are of knowing and addressing what needs attention at any given moment. Becker states, "It's important to remember that in every instance it is the process of attunement that is the point. The attainment, and the result it brings, is not something you should ever be concerned with. It is about attunement, not attainment. Beyond the attunement itself, everything else that takes place is simply a matter of expression; it is manifestation. This is a case of 'effects' again, and if you get hung up in that as attainment, then you have crossed your wires and you are back into the state of egotism."[177]

Our job is to settle under our own individual ego self needs and to allow ourselves to be guided by a mysterious intelligence beyond our ability to fully define, describe, or direct. When we learn to surrender to this profound force, we not only become a vehicle for the Breath of Life, but we also become available to receive its gifts directly. We may find our hearts opening with a sense of love pouring through us as we sit in awe of the healing process we, and our clients, witness together. We may also find we begin to live our lives differently.

A Biodynamic Curriculum

The curriculum for learning Craniosacral Biodynamics varies from school to school. The following is based on the curriculum developed and taught at Karuna Institute. It is also used at Stillpoint, a biodynamic school in New York City. Franklyn Sills has helped to establish Stillpoint, having trained the teachers while teaching a series of foundation trainings there. He continues to present at Stillpoint as a guest teacher, as well as teaching postgraduate seminars.

As mentioned earlier, the biodynamic practitioner training is usually at least two years in duration. During this time, trainees attend 350 hours of class and complete 350 hours of coursework between modules. Coursework at home includes about two practice sessions per week (totaling at least 150 practice sessions). Other coursework, taking approximately two or three hours per week, includes writeups of practice sessions to be turned in to tutors for feedback and supervision, written answers to questions which usually involve describing your own perceptual experience of specific skills being practiced and study of relevant anatomy. This usually involves drawing or tracing specific anatomical structures related to that module. In the second year, trainees complete a clinical project involving a course of ten practice sessions with two different clients, writeups of each session, and a brief research report on a medical condition one of these practice clients has. This clinical project is designed to help ground the skills learned in class and prepare the trainee for clinical practice.

The first year of the training is primarily oriented to supporting the profound perceptual shifts required in practicing this beautiful, subtle work. The second year takes trainees into more specific aspects of perception, including forces from the birth process and more skills in addressing unresolved traumatic experience arising in session work. Following is a module-by-module description of the curriculum.

Seminar One

In the first module, we take time to orient to the course and introduce ourselves. We begin with awareness and settling of the relational field, just as we would begin a session. We take time to discuss basic relational needs and how they can be met within the safe relational holding field of session work. We practice holding one another with a heart-centered sense of acceptance. We explore the felt sense of resource; begin mindfulness-based meditative practices; learn about establishing practitioner fulcrums enabling the practitioner to provide a safe, settled, grounded presence; and practice negotiating comfortable physical contact, as well as energetic distance between individuals. In this first seminar, we introduce the three bodies, physical, fluid, and tidal, and practice sensing them in our own systems through a "Three Body Chi Kung" practice. We introduce Primary Respiration, emphasizing fluid tide awareness, as it is a more embodied manifestation of Primary Respiration, supportive of staying grounded and present in relationship with each other, and is often easier to sense than long-tide phenomena. We begin with simple, safe contact at the feet, as well as some other holds to introduce cranial and sacral contact and practice listening skills. We also introduce dynamic stillness and supporting stillpoint—a gateway to stillness—as a way to enhance settling of an activated nervous system. We augment stillpoint by orienting to and resting in the pause of stillness that naturally occurs at the end of exhalation or inhalation in mid-tide. In this first seminar, we orient to exhalation stillpoint as it helps settle sympathetic activation. Inhalation stillpoints are more useful in states of dissociation and are taught later in the training.

Seminar Two

In seminar two, we review and continue deepening the skills introduced in the first seminar, including practicing tidal meditations. By this point, students are usually noticing a sense of settling in their practice sessions. As this is already being sensed, we introduce the Holistic Shift and its importance as a starting point. We introduce several cranial holds to give trainees a chance to develop ease of contacting them and begin to sense motility (movement of the tissues with the fluid tide) within the cranium. We begin to introduce the stress response, along with simple mindfulness-based verbal skills useful in supporting clients (and practitioners) in staying present in their bodies and in relationship when trauma arises. We introduce and practice verbal and trauma skills throughout the training.

Seminar Three

By the third seminar, students are usually beginning to experience increasing ease in perceiving at the fluid-tide level. By this point, they are often beginning to sense patterns in the tissues. We introduce the concept of organizing fulcrums, including natural biodynamic fulcrums, which Sutherland recognized as "automatically shifting" up and down the midline with the inhalation and exhalation of the tides. We also discuss inertial or conditional fulcrums resulting from various forces derived from life circumstances and traumas, and how these might be sensed. Even as we introduce the anatomy of the reciprocal tension membranes, we emphasize the importance in the biodynamic approach of orienting to what organizes the tissue patterns we perceive, rather staying at the level of the structural patterning. Sensing the patterns is useful in helping us find their fulcrums, but we are not trying to change the pattern. We introduce Becker's three-step process as a common expression of the inherent treatment plan at a fluid-tide level. We continue our work with mindfulness and trauma skills, including some basic neurobiology of the stress response and how to address hyper-arousal. By this point, though we have also introduced long tide and dynamic stillness, we continue to emphasize the grounding qualities of fluid tide. We also give the students extra feedback through hands-on tutorials. Each student listens to a tutor's system, with feedback on their contact as well as support in identifying what they are perceiving.

Seminar Four

By seminar four, most students are sensing fluid tide with some ease and beginning to develop awareness of stillness and long tide in their practice sessions. Having practiced being with Becker's three steps, they will have noticed that sometimes the system is unable to settle into a state of balance but continues seeking. Here we introduce skills of augmentation, which involve subtly enhancing the natural increasing of potency and space during inhalation of the fluid tide. This is a subtle breathing of our hands and awareness with inhalation. This is a skill that is not often required but can be useful in cases of extreme inertia where settling doesn't deepen. Students practice augmentation particularly in relation to the cranial bones and sutures. Usually by this point in the training, we also introduce images of embryological development to support therapeutic relationship to the fluid developmental forces expressing throughout life. We also continue developing verbal trauma skills and introduce concepts of transference and counter-transference as they can affect the relational field, including our ability to be present in a supportive way with the client. During seminars four and five, trainees engage in feedback sessions with the tutors, each student giving a tutor a session to demonstrate and receive support with specific basic skills practiced in the first few seminars. We also include relevant aspects of practice management, starting in the first module with the case study and including topics like how to introduce this work to a new or prospective client.

Seminar Five

In the fifth seminar, we introduce working with the vertebral column, including the pelvis. By this point in the training, when many trainees are more settled and subtle in their perception, we begin developing more long-tide skills. As a foundation for working with the boney midline of the spine, we first practice orienting to the primal midline, a long-tide phenomenon. Primal midline is the center of the bioelectric torus mentioned previously. It is the energetic path of the notochord, serving as an organizing fulcrum for essentially all body tissues both in the forming embryo and throughout life. Practitioner orientation to primal midline supports the client's system in reorienting to it where it has been distracted by unresolved conditional forces. We find awareness of primal midline may be occluded where there is holding due to past trauma or other unresolved events. As we hold the midline in relation to different vertebral structures and levels, we become aware of issues resolving and the midline clarifying. Before approaching specific vertebral structures with particular vertebral and cervical holds, we introduce listening to the connective tissue field as a whole in relation to primal midline. We can then add specific anatomical structures to our awareness.

Seminar Six

In seminar six, we introduce birth dynamics and explore cranial base patterns that often relate to birth. Here we introduce the spheno-basilar junction where the sphenoid and occiput meet as the site of an automatically, naturally shifting fulcrum for the bones. We listen to motility of the cranial base bones in relation to this central fulcrum and how other, inertial fulcrums affect the motility with cranial base patterning. We work with fulcrums presenting, supporting settling into a state of balance and resolution through Becker's three steps. We introduce birth dynamics, which often present in cranial base patterns. We practice verbal trauma skills related to dissociation and practice augmenting inhalation stillpoints, which can be helpful in dissociative states. Having begun the second year of the training, trainees at this point begin a clinical project. This involves working with at least two new clients for at least ten sessions each to experience continuity and how healing may evolve over a series of sessions. The project, completed between seminars six and nine, includes a short research paper on a clinical condition present in one of these project clients.

Seminar Seven

In seminar seven, we continue exploring the inherent treatment plan, now orienting to long tide as initiator of healing intentions. On a tissue level, we introduce transverse relationships (the pelvic and respiratory diaphragms, and thoracic inlet). We continue up the midline to work with the occipital triad (axis, atlas, and occiput), continuing to orient to primal midline in our session work. In this seminar, we also work with the central nervous system, as well as the nociceptive (pain- and danger-sensing) pathways, facilitation processes, and the brain stem. Facilitation refers to when nerve pathways become sensitized or overactive. In other words, their firing has become facilitated (made easier). This is common in chronic pain and often relates to an ongoing stress response, including the depression often accompanying chronic pain conditions. Along with relevant cranial methods, we also continue developing verbal trauma skills to help regulate an overactive stress response.

Seminar Eight

Continuing with our work with the nervous system, in this seminar we address the Polyvagal Theory and triune nervous system from the important work of Stephen Porges, and work specifically with the social engagement system. This works well with attending to relationships of the bones of the face, hard palate, and temporomandibular joint (TMJ). In relation to inertial fulcrums in these areas, we deepen skills of augmentation. This involves orienting to and breathing with the natural increase of potency within space with inhalation of the mid-tide. We continue practicing verbal trauma skills in relation to this nervous system and facial work. In seminars eight and nine, we have a second set of feedback sessions, where students give the tutors sessions, both for support in continuing to develop their skills and to evaluate if the student is on track for graduation in seminar ten.

Seminar Nine

In the ninth seminar, we review the central nervous system dynamics, polyvagal system, and include the hypothalamus-pituitary-adrenal (HPA) axis. We address the common occurrence of facilitation in this aspect of the stress response. We then address the organs, listening to the motility of the digestive organs, pelvic organs, and heart and lungs. This includes their common relationship to nociceptive facilitation introduced in seminar seven. In relation to heart motility, we also introduce the concept of ignition and work with augmenting heart ignition. Ignition refers to the starting up of the system at the end of each exhalation or beginning of each inhalation at the long-tide level. In the training, we explore three primary ignitions related to early development. Heart ignition relates to the important moment at just four weeks after conception when the heart begins beating. This time tends to coincide with when the parents discover the pregnancy or the pregnancy is confirmed. Any experience of ambivalence or outright rejection at this time can result in dampening of heart ignition, which tends to be reflected in energy levels and attitudes toward one's life and embodiment. Augmenting heart ignition can have profound effects on one's life and relationships, as well as heart function and motility. Throughout the training, we also continue to cover aspects of practice management in most modules. In this module, we usually introduce working with babies and children. Trainees interested in this area of work are encouraged to pursue postgraduate training to develop the special skills needed for working with little ones, particularly those who are preverbal.

Seminar Ten

It is always amazing to arrive at the end of a two-year training. Usually, tutors and trainees alike perceive profound changes in themselves and each other from the beginning of this journey together. Bonding over ten modules can be deep and touching, particularly in a residential training, like at Karuna. Seminar ten of course involves completions. As transitions, like completing a training, tend to reflect our birth experience, we find this is a good time to discuss prenatal and birth experience and how it potentially affects our psychology, our personality structure, relationship tendencies, beliefs, attitudes, and behaviors throughout life. In that the sense of this experience can arise during session work, we review this early experience from the perspective of the baby, and how easily shock and trauma can occur because of how the little one's nervous system functions. We continue with verbal and trauma skills useful with these issues. We also work with birth ignition, which relates to when the baby begins to breathe at birth and the umbilical cord stops pulsing. If, as is so common in modern Western birth practices, the umbilical cord is cut before it stops pulsing, this ignition can be dampened. Augmenting umbilical ignition can support one's sense of empowerment to be an individual living one's own life. We also work with conception ignition, relating to the moment of conception. Issues around belonging and wanting to be here on earth can be addressed through augmenting conception ignition, which can be dampened by the environment we find ourselves coming into, or our own karmic influences that we bring with us into this life. Following these subtle yet profound sessions, we address any important practice management issues that have not already been covered, such as supervision and postgraduate options. We then move into celebration mode!

As you read this, you are most likely in an early stage of learning about Craniosacral Biodynamics. The next chapter, "Resources for Learning More," includes information about biodynamic associations, relevant reading and other media, as well as options for postgraduate studies in case you have already completed or are completing the foundation training. Guidance for completing prerequisites to the practitioner training is also included, such as anatomy and physiology courses.

9
Resources for Learning More

This chapter is primarily provided as a reference to support you in your next steps. While the previous chapter discusses finding a biodynamic practitioner and receiving sessions, which are highly recommended before applying for biodynamic training, this chapter begins with guidance for fulfilling other prerequisites to the training. This is followed by a section on options for postgraduate work, which includes complementary areas of study, such as trauma therapy and prenatal and birth therapy. The chapter concludes with a list of relevant readings and other media, as well as other resources to support you on your biodynamic journey.

Moving toward Training: Fulfilling Prerequisites

Once you have received biodynamic sessions and decided this is something you want to learn to practice, the next step is to look into available trainings. As mentioned in the previous chapter, schools and teachers are listed on the websites of their biodynamic associations. I encourage you to explore these websites and discover what or whom you are drawn to. You may, however, be reading this book because you have "stumbled upon" or been mysteriously drawn to a biodynamic practitioner and have already decided you want to study at the school they graduated from. It is not unusual for people to find themselves intuitively drawn to a training, often without knowing much about the work they are about to immerse themselves in. If this applies to you, know that you are in good company!

Whatever your path to your training, it can be helpful to find out what is required of those applying for the training. Most trainings require that you have a minimum number of hours of coursework in general anatomy and physiology. These can often be acquired through an online course, as well as by attending classes in person.

Usually, you will be interviewed before being accepted to your training. The tutors interviewing you will be assessing your ability to participate and manage what the training entails. This includes practical issues, like being able to afford tuition and pay it in a timely fashion. Because the training can be challenging, it is important that you have a certain degree of grounding and stability in your own life, and are not already overwhelmed by stress or your own history. In this vein, you may be recommended to undergo a series of biodynamic sessions or a course of psychotherapy or trauma therapy before beginning the training. These are also often recommended as adjuncts to the training.

As previously mentioned, most trainings also require or give preference to applicants who are already practitioners of some kind. If you are not already trained or practicing some kind of therapy, your first step before the biodynamic training may be fulfilling that prerequisite. Often prospective biodynamic trainees take a massage therapy course prior to Craniosacral Biodynamics as a relatively quick way to prepare for the training. While massage is a different modality, the specifics of anatomy and skills involved in touch can be very useful background for studying Craniosacral Biodynamics, as well as leading to a professional license to touch. Such a course will usually also provide sufficient hours in anatomy and physiology to meet that prerequisite for the biodynamic training.

Other areas of study that can be useful, although not required before starting a biodynamic training, are trauma therapies and mindfulness practices. These are expanded on further in the next section on postgraduate options.

Continuing and Deepening the Biodynamic Journey: Postgraduate Options

Completing the foundation training in Craniosacral Biodynamics enables you to begin professionally practicing this profound work. It can be helpful, however, to remember that it is designed to provide a *foundation* upon which to develop and deepen your practice.

As I witness trainees graduating in seminar ten of the training, I am often reminded of my own experience after completing my degree in occupational therapy. Although the training had included many hours of clinical experience in a variety of settings, when I started my first real job as an occupational therapist, I realized there was more to learn on the job than I had actually learned in the training. I think this is probably true for most occupations, Craniosacral Biodynamics included. When I was taking the foundation training myself, I remember thinking this was one thing I would never stop studying. There are so many layers and subtleties to this work! William Sutherland, the original pioneer in Cranial Osteopathy who set the stage for our work, practiced for forty years. As far as I can tell, he never stopped learning. His perception continued to deepen and develop throughout his life. I feel this is similar to my path in Craniosacral Biodynamics. Every session is a new experience. I am repeatedly surprised and awed by what arises in sessions, by what is possible to perceive, and by the Intelligence of the potency of the Breath of Life in action. I expect this will continue as long as I am able to continue practicing.

This is perhaps a long-winded way to recommend postgraduate studies and activities. The foundation training is just the beginning, a portal to a profound journey that potentially lasts a lifetime. The information in this section is to guide you in continuing your voyage.

A relatively simple way to continue your biodynamic studies after graduation is to take postgraduate seminars. The school you trained at probably offers such seminars. Following are some possibilities for postgraduate studies specifically in Craniosacral Biodynamics, as well as more in-depth studies in related areas of trauma therapy, prenatal and birth psychology and therapy, embryology, and mindfulness meditation. Apart from the specific biodynamic postgraduate seminars, these can be taken as preparation for the Craniosacral Biodynamics training or after graduation. Supervision and psychotherapy are also discussed as important adjuncts to practicing Craniosacral Biodynamics.

Postgraduate Seminars Offered at Karuna and around the World

Many schools offering a foundation training in Craniosacral Biodynamics also host postgraduate seminars. These may be designed specifically for graduates of Craniosacral Biodynamics trainings, or may be open to cranial practitioners with non-biodynamic backgrounds. At Karuna, we offer postgraduate seminars covering many topics. Most of our seminars are five days; some are three or four. If you are a cranial practitioner wanting to include a biodynamic approach, or if you are looking to review, clarify, and deepen your understanding and practice of Craniosacral Biodynamics, we recommend beginning with our course Breath of Life: The Three Bodies and the Three Functions of

Potency. In this seminar, we review the essentials of the three bodies and Primary Respiration, including settling of the relational field with heart-centered presence, the holistic shift, inherent treatment plan in relation to functions of potency, and dynamic stillness. We offer other biodynamic seminars, emphasizing prenatal and birth influences, verbal and hands-on trauma skills and the neurobiology of trauma, working with ignition processes, visceral work, and the long tide. Other postgraduate seminars we offer include: Awakening the Heart, The Primal Midline, The Three Functions of Potency, and Brain, Heart and Being. Franklyn Sills and I coteach most of these seminars around Europe and North America, as well as at Karuna. As of this writing, we are cutting back on travel and developing an online school, www.resourcingyourlife.org, which will also offer biodynamic courses.

Other biodynamic schools offer a variety of postgraduate seminars. As mentioned in chapter 7, you can find a list of biodynamic schools at the website for the International Affiliation of Biodynamic Trainings (IABT) at http://biodynamic-craniosacral.org or www.iabt.org. Some schools also offer seminars in related topics, like embryology or trauma skills. The next section covers separate seminars and trainings in complementary areas.

Studies, Training, and Experiential Seminars in Complementary Areas

As you have seen, the practice of Craniosacral Biodynamics is greatly supported by our ability to be present to generate a safe relational field. This is facilitated through our own practices in presence, as well as our understanding and healing in relation to our own trauma histories, including early prenatal and birth experience. This section offers some suggestions for furthering your studies in these areas.

Trauma therapy is a very popular field these days. As well as specific biodynamic seminars to deepen your skills in working with trauma, there are a large variety of seminars and trainings available. One of the most well-known is in Somatic Experiencing (SE), the approach to trauma developed by Peter Levine. There are SE trainings available all over the world, as well as certified practitioners you can work with to help you develop skills and address your own trauma history. The SE training is composed of six seminars, generally offered over three years. You can learn more about these trainings and find practitioners in your area at the SE website at www.sosinternationale.org.

Apart from a full SE training or working with a practitioner, there are several excellent sources of information about trauma therapy available online and around the world. One of my favorites is the National Institute for the Clinical Application of Behavioral Medicine (NICABM), hosted by psychologist Ruth Buczynski. At their website, www.nicabm.com, NICABM offers online interviews and short courses with specialists in the field of trauma therapy, neurobiology, and research. Many of the NICABM programs are available free of charge for a short time, or recordings can be accessed at your convenience for a reasonable fee. Presenters on trauma include Bessel van der Kolk, Peter Levine, Ruth Lanius, Dan Siegel, and Stephen Porges, all of whom have written books I recommend in relation to your biodynamic journey. (For recommended reading and viewing, please see the list at the end of this chapter.)

NICABM also provides programs on mindfulness as applied to psychotherapy and trauma therapy, which is highly relevant to our work with Craniosacral Biodynamics. These often include the research in the neurobiology of mindfulness. There are important overlaps between trauma therapy and mindfulness meditation. In contemporary trauma therapy research, orienting to sensations in present time has been found to be essential to shifting neural pathways involved in trauma responses and PTSD. Mindfulness practices enhance functions in brain areas related to present time orientation, integration, and meaning making, all of which can be interrupted by unresolved trauma and a chronically overactive stress response.

As well as learning about the value and integration of mindfulness practices into any kind of therapy through NICABM and other courses and readings, biodynamic practice can be supported by deepening your own mindfulness practices. There are many choices available here. Eight-week mindfulness courses are offered around the world by instructors trained in mindfulness-based stress reduction (MBSR). This represents the work of Jon Kabat-Zinn, who has applied aspects of more traditional Vipassana meditation in medical and mental health settings. Meditation retreats of various lengths are also available for developing and deepening your mindfulness practice. Vipassana meditation involves honing your skills in attending to breath and sensations in a mindful way. Courses are available through Insight Meditation (www.insightmeditation.org) and Vipassana (www.dhamma.org). The Vietnamese Buddhist monk Thich Nhat Hanh has also taught mindfulness meditation around the world, including at his retreat center, Plum Village, in France. Courses in this style can be found at https://plumvillage.org. There are many inspiring books written by Thich Nhat Hanh, as well as by teachers of Vipassana, like Tara Brach, Joseph Goldstein, and Jack Kornfield.

Another training including mindfulness is the Core Process Psychotherapy training, originally developed by Maura Sills with the support of Franklyn Sills. This is a psychotherapy training based on Buddhist principles of presence, offering skills in mindfulness-based psychotherapy and trauma resolution, including an introduction to prenatal and birth trauma. If you are already a practitioner of some sort, including if you have completed a biodynamic training, you can take a part-time two-year postqualifications master's degree at Karuna, or you can take the longer three-year Core Process clinical training. Each can be followed up by a clinical year to become an accredited psychotherapist (within the UK; check requirements for other regions).

Prenatal and Birth Psychology and Therapy

Prenatal and birth psychology and therapy is another field essential to any study and healing of trauma. While you may be unaware of your own prenatal or birth history having been in any way traumatic, wounding in this early time of life is widespread and often not in our conscious awareness. Our bodies, however, hold our memories of this time, and our history tends to be expressed through our behaviors, relationships, and tendencies. These are particularly apparent when we are in transition or starting something new, such as you moving into learning about or practicing Craniosacral Biodynamics.

As you will see in reading about supervision, issues involved in starting a biodynamic practice may stem from very early experience, such as when we were in the womb or being born, as well as from postnatal and childhood events. Similarly, our cranial and somatic patterning, ways of holding tension, and nervous system activation tendencies may have been established in this early, preverbal period. While receiving biodynamic sessions can help resolve these issues, learning about prenatal and birth experience, and its associated psychology, can be immensely helpful in enhancing awareness of this territory, and how to be with it. Working with a prenatal and birth-oriented therapist can be extremely supportive. Exploring this material in workshops or small groups can also be very effective in healing, as can learning about the consciousness and challenges of this time of life.

When we have very early trauma, it is common to not be consciously aware of its influence or even its occurrence. While there is now ample evidence that babies, even before birth, are highly sentient, aware beings, the common attitude toward little ones before, during, and after birth is that they are cute and cuddly little things to be kept clean, fed, and as quiet as possible. Their feelings about what is happening to them are rarely considered or addressed, although fortunately awareness of the intelligent sentience of babies is increasing. Those involved in the field of prenatal and birth psychology work hard to reveal and disseminate evidence of awareness, memory, learning, and intelligence in little ones before they are born and through the months following birth. Babies are gradually being treated with increasing respect but insensitive, rough handling and quick, often unnecessary birth interventions continue to be practiced without communication with the very present, potentially cooperative baby.

Babies process stimuli more slowly than you and me, as everything is new to their developing brains and nervous systems. They respond well to slow, gentle handling, with simple explanations as to what is about to happen and why. Although we don't understand how they seem to understand the words spoken to them, they clearly respond appropriately and intelligently when given the chance. For example, babies can cooperate by turning when someone explains to them the consequences of their position before birth and that they just need to move a little in a particular direction to avoid a cesarean section. Babies are hard-wired at birth for social communication. Their social engagement nervous system is online. They may be more interested in gazing into Mom's eyes than in finding her breast and feeding. They certainly respond to tone of voice and levels of activity around them. Babies can be shocked by arriving into a brightly lit room with many strangers presenting masks instead of faces, all moving in an accelerated, urgent fashion, often involving physical pain to the little one.

There are many simple and complex events and stimuli that can be traumatizing for babies at birth. My intention here is not to enumerate every possible form of birth trauma, but to emphasize how experiencing them may influence our perception, behavior, personality, and tendencies throughout life. Having awareness of these kinds of experiences can be a major first step toward resolving or at least managing them. As with any trauma, our history does not go away when we work with it, but our relationship to it can change dramatically. This can be liberating in many ways, and can support our ability to be present and compassionate with our clients, as well as ourselves and others in our lives.

One important aspect of prenatal, birth, and other preverbal trauma is that it is usually not recorded in our conscious, verbal memory. When we are unaware of it, we tend to act it out unconsciously, repeatedly experiencing ourselves as victims powerless to effect change in our environment, dependent on a doctor to pull us out of the womb or to get us breathing, metaphorically speaking. This early experience becomes a major aspect of our unconscious shadow material until we develop awareness of it.

Resolving this early trauma usually also requires experiencing a different, more sensitive and nurturing kind of holding field. Again, biodynamic sessions can provide this, but there may be more healing and awareness available through specifically addressing this time of life.

There are several ways to learn more about this time of life and begin to shift our relationship with our own early history. As mentioned previously, working with a prenatal- and birth-oriented therapist can be helpful. Practitioners in this area are listed on the website for the Association for Prenatal and Perinatal Psychology and Health (APPPAH) at www.birthpsychology.com. APPPAH has also recently established an online prenatal and birth education program. This is an excellent way to intellectually learn more about this time of life and to begin exploring your relationship with it. There are also numerous books on the topic, some of which are listed at the end of this chapter. APPPAH also has an extensive reading list available on their website.

More experiential approaches are generally essential in order to shift your own early imprints and perception, enabling you to be more fully present with your clients' issues when they arise. The most effective approach I have encountered for working with this material is the small womb surround process workshops developed by Raymond Castellino (www.castellinotraining.com). These small groups are usually made up of three to eight participants and one or two assistants, as well as the facilitator. Each participant has a turn during the workshop during which the entire group supports him or her in addressing their intention. Castellino has meticulously developed a workshop structure designed to establish safety and support for each member of the group, while regulating nervous system activation, which is so important in resolving trauma. These groups can be an excellent way to both heal and learn about early trauma. In leading these small womb surround process workshops, I usually find myself witnessing and facilitating profound life-changing healing and insights among the participants.

Another pioneer in the field of prenatal and birth psychology, William Emerson offers larger seminars where participants usually work in pairs or groups of three, supported by Emerson and assistants, to explore their early history. Emerson uses guided regression (or egression) methods, and includes exploration of spiritual dimensions of coming into a life. Emerson's website is http://emersonbirthrx.com.

Both Emerson and Castellino offer training for practitioners intending to practice prenatal and birth therapy, or to integrate this perspective into their work. Having personally studied extensively with both of these pioneers in the field, I can recommend their work as helpful for developing skill and insight in relation to this early material.

Another option for learning more about prenatal and birth trauma and how to work with it is offered by Franklyn Sills and me through the Karuna Institute. Our Prenatal Person training is a six-module training for practitioners (http://karuna-institute.co.uk /prenatal-person.html). We also offer postgraduate seminars related to embryological influences and prenatal and birth issues that may arise in biodynamic sessions. Our new online school (www.resourcingyourlife.org) will also offer webinars and courses in prenatal and birth psychology, mindfulness-based trauma skills, Craniosacral Biodynamics, and Continuum to somatically inquire into these areas (more information on Continuum follows).

Embryology

Related to prenatal and birth experience, one other option helpful in deepening into Craniosacral Biodynamics is to learn about embryology. Embryological development is both fascinating and highly relevant to Craniosacral Biodynamics. The biodynamic forces we work with are equally active in forming the embryo and in us throughout our lives. In Craniosacral Biodynamics sessions, we find that as the system resolves inertial issues, potency can shift from its protective and then healing function to its organizational function. Here, we often perceive the client as reforming according to the original blueprint affecting our original formation as embryos. We may feel as if we are holding a little one, as the cells and tissues orient toward the primal midline. Understanding embryological development can help us to be with the unfolding process in the client, including any trauma related to early developmental issues in the womb or at birth, and the reorganization as old issues resolve.

My favorite embryologist to study with is Jaap van der Wal. His background steeped in Steiner (whose ideas inspired Steiner or Waldorf education and biodynamic farming) and Gautian philosophy infuses his teachings with a spiritual quality unusual in embryology. He is also a wonderful storyteller, which is useful when spending hours listening to tales of how we develop in the womb! Van der Wal offers workshops around the world. His schedule as well as several excellent articles and wonderful images are available at his website, www.embryo.nl. More details on embryology resources are available at the end of this chapter.

On a more somatic level, I also offer workshops exploring embryology through Continuum around the world. These Embodying Embryology workshops involve learning about aspects of embryological development through PowerPoint presentations, along with experiential explorations using the breaths, sounds, subtle movement, and awareness of Continuum. I find this an amazing way to access what I call our original embryological potential, because we so easily and naturally enter into primordial, fluidic states, like those of the embryo, in Continuum.

Continuum and Other Somatic Movement Practices

Continuum, developed by the late Emilie Conrad over almost fifty years, continues to evolve through a dedicated community of teachers and practitioners (www .continuumteachers.com). This profound somatic practice is extremely complementary to Craniosacral Biodynamics. Using specific breaths, vocalized sounds, both intentional and spontaneous movement, and mindful awareness, Continuum takes us into similar perceptual territories as Craniosacral Biodynamics. I often use it as a teaching tool in my biodynamic classes to support students in experiencing biodynamic concepts, as well as anatomy and embryology, within their own bodies. Like Craniosacral Biodynamics, Continuum facilitates slowing down and settling under everyday and historical patterning, deepening into peaceful, resourcing fluidic states. In Continuum, we often experience ourselves as moving, floating, and being like a liquid embryo within the womb, as with the fluid body in Craniosacral Biodynamics. Or we may feel as if we are suspended in a spacious cosmic field, similar to the biodynamic perception of long tide.

Because of its emphasis on sensory perception and mindful awareness of the body, its movement, sensations, and patterning, I tend to see Continuum as a somatic mindfulness practice. Like other mindfulness practices, I find Continuum can be helpful for resolving trauma because of how it slows our pacing and helps regulate the nervous system. It also introduces delicious, pleasurable sensations, which can become a nurturing resource, supporting resilience. A major effect of very early trauma is resistance to entering our bodies, avoiding fully embodied living. Continuum can challenge this tendency by enhancing sensory experience, with a mindful observation that enhances our ability to be with whatever we may be experiencing.

Many of my Continuum workshops also involve some aspects of accessing early embryological developmental potential. These workshops are not designed as a way to explore your trauma, but can support healing issues from this early time by enhancing awareness and enabling us to access the original potential interrupted by our trauma.

As mentioned, Continuum is also an excellent adjunct to Craniosacral Biodynamics, often referred to as a way to give ourselves Craniosacral Biodynamicd sessions. It naturally takes us into similar states as Craniosacral Biodynamics and can have similarly beneficial effects. One of the postgraduate seminars I offer, called Embodying

Biodynamics, presents important Craniosacral Biodynamics principles explored both through Continuum and table sessions.

Other movement and somatic practices can also be supportive of your biodynamic journey. There are too many to list all here, but may include tai chi and chi kung, yoga, body-mind centering (BMC), and somatic psychotherapy.

Supervision as a Path of Healing, Learning, and Support

Many practitioners new to Craniosacral Biodynamics are surprised to learn that supervision is highly recommended and often required for registration. In other forms of bodywork, supervision is often seen as useful to support technical skills or, perhaps, in cases of sexual attraction to a client. Certainly, supervision can be supportive in these ways. For a highly relational practice like Craniosacral Biodynamics, however, it is essential.

We have explored in earlier chapters how integral the relational field is in biodynamic session work. Clients need to feel safe enough for their nervous system to deepen under defensive modes, enabling the holistic shift to occur and potency to shift from its defensive to healing functions. Where the relationship between client and practitioner is primary, relational issues tend to arise. It is not unusual for clients to perceive the practitioner as if they were someone from the client's past. Known as "transference" in psychodynamic therapies, this usually involves the client reacting to the therapist as if they were an authority figure from the past, often a parent, teacher, religious leader, or even a previous therapist. In that therapists are also human, carrying their own history, they may react to the client's transference or perceive the client as someone from their own history. This is known as counter-transference. These dynamics can be confusing and challenging, as well as potentially very healing. In one of the few books about Craniosacral Therapy written by women, craniosacral therapists Liz Kalinowska and Daska Hatton write, "An awareness of the concepts of transference and counter-transference is even more important for bodywork practitioners than it is for traditional talk-based psychotherapists, as the additional stimulus of touch and the felt sense adds more potential difficulties to negotiate."[178]

In that transference and counter-transference are usually unconscious phenomena, they typically require an outside witness to enable awareness and clarity of what is happening and to prevent potentially harmful, unconscious acting out of the past. Supervision is important as an additional field of support within which session work can safely and ethically unfold.

Because supervision is not highly valued in most bodywork practices, there is often misunderstanding or lack of knowledge as to its purpose. New graduates may resent a requirement for supervision, not valuing what it can contribute to their practice. So, what is supervision, and why is it important?

What Is Supervision and Why Do We Need It?

Supervision involves meeting with a supervisor, preferably on a regular basis, to discuss and explore issues arising for the practitioner in session work. Supervisors are not necessarily trained or experienced in Craniosacral Biodynamics, although this may be useful and may be required by your regulating agency. It is important that supervisors have training and experience in holding personal process. They may have training in psychotherapy and trauma therapy, as well as specific training in supervision. The intention of supervision is to support the practitioner in being able to be present with clients, particularly when challenging situations arise. While it may cover similar territories to psychotherapy, and at times may resemble psychotherapy, it differs from psychotherapy in its intention. The central focus of supervision is what benefits the supervisee's clients, whereas for psychotherapy it is what benefits the psychotherapy client. In that our clients benefit from our enhanced clarity with our own issues, supervision may look like sessions primarily about these issues.

Many kinds of challenges can present in session work for practitioners with any amount of experience. For new practitioners, support may be around developing confidence as a practitioner, being with doubts, fears, and insecurities around trusting what happens in a session, as well as in being able to put themselves out to the public through advertising, networking, etc. I love supervising new practitioners because I find it often becomes obvious that they are moving through a birth process, one of my favorite things to be with.

Starting a new career and a new practice is a new beginning in life. As such, it is a momentous occasion, likely to echo one's birth experience. Where birth was easy and the person felt safe and welcomed in the process, entering into a new practice may be similarly easy and flowing. For many of us, birth was not so ideal, and new beginnings or transitions in life tend to rekindle unfinished business from that time. New practitioners may feel unworthy, feeling they do not deserve to charge for their services. Or they may feel vulnerable in advertising their services, holding back or procrastinating due to old feelings of needing to hide in order to stay safe. They may have difficulty setting boundaries, such as limiting the duration of the session to the agreed-upon time. Practitioners at any stage in their practice may have a tendency to placate their clients, needing to be liked, fearing they will not return, or that others will discover how incompetent they are. Or they may be driven by a need to fix their clients, making their pain and suffering go away. Any of these issues can reflect aspects of the psyche that can benefit from nonjudgmental acknowledgment, empathy, and holding, as well as interfering with listening to and trusting the unfolding of the inherent treatment plan.

Challenges with establishing a new practice frequently mirror very early issues relating to a deep, even unconscious sense of worthiness, ability to progress, step out on your own, and be seen, be independent. These issues can relate to very early experience, such as how it was to have your existence discovered when you were in the womb, how it was to have your gender discovered before or at birth, how nourished and supported you felt in the womb, during, or after birth, as well as how you were seen, heard, respected, received, and appreciated as a child. While psychotherapy can be useful and may be essential in addressing these issues, supervision can also be supportive in bringing them to light, and helping establish a different kind of holding field for you as you venture out into the world in a new way.

If you consider that starting a new practice in a new field, particularly with a new paradigm, is a form of birth, you are birthing yourself into a new life. You deserve to be supported in this journey. You particularly need support if that is a foreign concept for you! So many practitioners are far better at providing support to others than at receiving it themselves. As you have probably learned by now from earlier discussion in this book, and perhaps from your experience so far with Craniosacral Biodynamics, this work has so much to do with receiving. This may be part of the paradigm shift for you. Please allow yourself to be supported in this process!

Even if the challenges mentioned don't arise, it is important to acknowledge that clients bring their pain and share their suffering with us. Our work can be intense at times. It can be a lot to hold our clients' processes on our own. In that our work is held in confidentiality to protect our clients, we can't just go home and talk to our spouse or friends about what happened in a session on a particularly overwhelming day. Supervision is there to support us in these situations. When we have regular supervision, we establish a trusting relationship with a supervisor we feel safe with, where we can be held and can have extra holding for our clients.

I see supervision as an important aspect of our ability in Craniosacral Biodynamics to rest into fields within fields of support. Consider the cellular-tissue field of the physical body as suspended within the fluid field, suspended within the tidal body of long tide, and all of this suspended within the supportive field of supervision. To me, this is similar to how little ones need to be held early in life. The baby is held by the mother, who is supported by her partner, both of whom are supported by their family, birth assistants, and community. Without these fields of support, mothers often become overly stressed and can easily be overwhelmed. The little one she holds is also affected by the lack of support. Unfortunately, this scenario is far too common in our modern world, where social isolation, as well as isolation during the birth process, is not unusual. We find that, when mothers receive the support they need, common mother-baby issues resolve remarkably easily. For example, when a new baby is having trouble latching onto the breast and feeding, it is not unusual for this to shift dramatically by just holding the mother and helping her to feel safe and settle into holistic shift. Similarly, our clients often settle more deeply and easily when we, as practitioners, receive the support we need.

In recognition of supervision as an important adjunct to practicing Craniosacral Biodynamics, some registration agencies have supervision requirements. For example, the CSTA in both the UK and BCTA in North America have a minimal requirement for supervision. In the UK, this requirement is four sessions per year, or eight sessions over two years, for the first two years of practice after graduation. The North American association has had a similar requirement, although it now includes personal growth activities that support the practitioner in being able to be more present with their clients in the face of challenging interpersonal issues that may arise. These include process-oriented workshops, such as prenatal and birth-process workshops, as well as psychotherapy or other process-oriented group sessions like family constellations work.

While such work can help practitioners in being clearer about when their own unresolved history is being touched by a relationship with a client, I still see ongoing supervision as essential for support. Because of the relationship established between practitioner and supervisor, profound healing can occur, as can the possibility of resting into an external field of support. I highly recommend having ongoing, regular supervision with someone you feel comfortable with so as to have someone available to take your issues to as they arise. I find that having ongoing supervision, even after years of practice, keeps me curious. Even if I don't have many challenges these days with my client work, I find I observe myself in my work with consideration for how my supervisor might perceive the situation or where I might grow further. Supervision, like psychotherapy, has the potential to enable further growth and development. Remember that development is about meeting new challenges. Having support available for when these arise facilitates meeting and learning from what challenges us, rather than either being overwhelmed or missing the opportunity by being dismissive. Just as useful as the support for our insecurities is the nudge to awaken and breathe where we are holding, and to open to discovery where we are arrogant.

It has become very clear to me through my study and practice of Craniosacral Biodynamics that it is a field in which learning and growth can continue ad infinitum. This realization is actually part of what inspired me to train to teach this profound work. I had passed through so many practices that I found myself growing out of. Craniosacral Biodynamics felt like something I would never grow tired of, would never fully comprehend, and would never stop being challenged and supported by. I hope you will also join the call of this path of health and healing, if you feel so moved. I look forward to meeting you in the field.

> Somewhere out beyond our sense
> Of right doing and wrong doing
> There is a field … I'll meet you there.
>
> —*Rumi*

For Further Reading, Listening, and Watching

While there are increasing resources available online and in print, here are some suggestions for getting started.

Craniosacral Biodynamics

Menzam-Sills, Cherionna. *The Breath of Life.* Recordings of guided explorations from this book available at http://www.birthingyourlife.org/the-breath-of-life-book/.

Sills, Franklyn. *Foundations in Craniosacral Biodynamics, Volumes 1 and 2.*

Sills, Franklyn. *Craniosacral Biodynamics: Foundations and Core Principles,* DVD series, available from Whole Being Films. http://wholebeingfilms.com/.

Trauma, Development, and Interpersonal Neurobiology

Badenoch, Bonnie. *Being a Brain-Wise Therapist: A Practical Guide to Neurobiology.*

Levine, Peter. *An Unspoken Voice.*

NICABM. www.nicabm.com.

Porges, Stephen. http://stephenporges.com.

Sensorimotor Psychotherapy, developed by Pat Ogden and others. https://www.senso-rimotorpsychotherapy.org.

Sills, Franklyn. *Being and Becoming: Psychodynamics, Buddhism, and the Origins of Selfhood.*

Sills, Franklyn. *Craniosacral Biodynamics: Foundations and Core Principles*, DVD series, available from Whole Being Films. http://wholebeingfilms.com/.

Somatic Experiencing, the work of Peter Levine. https://traumahealing.org.

Van der Kolk, Bessel. *The Body Keeps the Score: Mind, Brain and Body in the Transformation of Trauma.*

Mindfulness

Brach, Tara. https://www.tarabrach.com.

Insight Meditation. http://www.insightmeditation.org.

Kabat-Zinn, Jon. *Full Catastrophe Living: How to Cope with Stress, Pain and Illness Using Mindfulness Meditation.*

NICABM. www.nicabm.com.

Thich Nhat Han. https://plumvillage.org.

Vipassana. www.dhamma.org.

Anatomy and Physiology

Acland, Robert. *Acland's Video Atlas of Human Anatomy.*

Netter, Frank H. *Atlas of Human Anatomy.*

Clemente, Carmine D. *Anatomy: A Regional Atlas of the Human Body.*

Nolte, John. *The Human Brain.*

Paulsen, Friedrich, and Jens Waschke. *Sobotta Atlas of Human Anatomy.*

Wilsen-Pawels, Linda, et al. *Cranial Nerves.*

Embryology

Blechschmidt, Erich, and Raymond F. Gasser. *Biokinetics and Biodynamics of Human Differentiation: Principles and Applications.*

Blechschmidt, Erich, and Raymond F. Gasser. *The Ontogenetic Basis of Human Anatomy: A Biodynamic Approach to Development from Conception to Birth.*

Schoenworlf, Gary C., Steven B. Bleyl, Philip R. Brauer, and Philippa H. Francis-West. *Larsen's Embryology.*

Van der Wal, Jaap. Excellent articles and DVDs available on his website as well as his worldwide teaching schedule. http://www.embryo.nl.

Prenatal and Birth Psychology and Therapy

Association for Prenatal and Perinatal Psychology and Health. An excellent source of information on the field of prenatal and birth psychology, includes online courses, conferences, and reading lists. www.birthpsychology.com.

Emerson Seminars. Website of Prenatal and Birth Therapy pioneer William R. Emerson. http://emersonbirthrx.com.

Ray Castellino Trainings. Includes womb surround process workshops and training. www.castellinotraining.com.

Other Useful Websites

Karuna Institute. http://www.karuna-institute.co.uk.

Menzam-Sills, Cherionna. Website and blog. www.birthingyourlife.org.
Video blog: birthingyourlife.blogspot.co.uk.
Blog: cherionna.blogspot.co.uk.

Pacific Distributing Books & Bones. Distributes cranial and osteopathic-related books and supplies. https://www.booksandbones.com.

Resourcing Your Life. Online school of Franklyn Sills and Cherionna Menzam-Sills. www.resourcingyourlife.org.

Sills, Franklyn. Website. http://www.craniosacral-biodynamics.org.

Stillpoint Biodynamic school in New York City. Franklyn Sills helped establish this school, designed the curriculum for it, and continues to supervise and guest teach there. www.stillpointcst.com.

Biodynamic or Craniosacral Therapy Associations

These include practitioner listings as well as information about training to become a practitioner. Some countries have specific biodynamic associations. Others have umbrella Craniosacral Therapy associations in which Craniosacral Biodynamics is included.

International Affiliation of Biodynamic Trainings (IABT): Organization of trainings, includes list of graduates from each school (note that graduates may or may not be practicing). http://biodynamic-craniosacral.org.

Australia/New Zealand/Asia/Canada: Pacific Association of Craniosacral Therapists (PACT). Supports biodynamic practitioners with a list of practitioners and information on training to become one. http://www.bcst.info.

Austria: Cranio Austria: Austrian Federation for Craniosacral Work. An umbrella organization including biodynamic practitioners and trainings.

Belgium: International CranioSacral Association (ICSA). Umbrella organization including biodynamic practitioners. http://www.icsa-belgium.be.

Denmark: Foreningen Af Kranio-Sacral Terapeuter. Umbrella organization including biodynamic practitioners. http://www.kstforeningen.dk/.

France: Association Française de Thérapie Crânio-Sacrale Biodynamique (AFTCSB). http://www.therapiecraniosacrale.fr.

Germany: Craniosacral Verband Deutschland. Umbrella organization including biodynamically oriented schools and practitioners. http://www.cranioverband.org/.

Ireland: Irish Association of Craniosacral Therapists (IACST). Umbrella association including biodynamic practitioners. http://www.iacst.ie.

Italy: Associazione Craniosacrale Italia. http://www.acsicraniosacrale.it.

Netherlands: There are several organizations that include Craniosacral Biodynamics:

1. NCSV: the Nederlandse Cranio Sacraal Vereniging. www.cranio-sacraal.org. Union for Craniosacral therapists primarily trained through PCSA, the

Peirsman Cranio Sacral Academie, www.pcsa.nu; they embrace Craniosacral Biodynamics.

2. RCN: Register Craniosacraal Therapeuten in Nederland. www.register-rcn.nl. Union for qualified craniosacral therapists who mainly got their training in de UIN, the Upledger Instituut Nederland, www.upledger.nl. The RCN has started embracing Craniosacral Biodynamics, including accrediting biodynamic courses.

3. UCN: Upledger Craniosacraal Therapie Nederland. www.ucncranio.nl. Professional union of Upledger Cranio-Sacral therapists. They have organized introductory seminars in Craniosacral Biodynamics, with Franklyn Sills or senior tutors trained at Karuna.

Russia: Russian Craniosacral Academy. At the time of publication, a Russian Association of Craniosacral Biodynamics is being developed. http://cranio-acad.ru.

South Africa: Craniosacral Therapy Association of South Africa. An umbrella association including biodynamic approaches. http://www.cranial.org.za.

Spain: Asociación Española de Terapia Biodinámica Craneosacral (AETBC). http://www.asociacioncraneosacral.com.

Switzerland: Cranio Suisse, The Swiss Society for Craniosacral Therapy. Umbrella association including biodynamically oriented schools and practitioners. http://www.craniosuisse.ch. Since September, 2015, Craniosacral Therapy has been recognized as a method of Complimentary Therapy. As such, practitioners are required to have a specific medical background to practice. Information on schools and requirements is available on this website. There is also a website for the new Swiss federal diploma, called Complementary Therapist, specialization in Craniosacral-Therapie: www.oda-kt.ch.

United Kingdom: Craniosacral Therapy Association (CSTA). UK-based organization, umbrella association including but not limited to biodynamic practitioners and trainings. http://www.craniosacral.co.uk.

United States and Canada: Biodynamic Craniosacral Therapy Association of North America. www.craniosacraltherapy.org.

United States/Oregon: Northwest Cranial Association. Association for cranial practitioners with different backgrounds work to meet, support, and learn from each other and to promote public awareness. http://nwcranial.com.

Craniosacral Therapy Associations and Regulating Agencies

Graduates of biodynamic trainings may be eligible for registration with regulating agencies in their local area. These organizations are not necessarily biodynamically oriented, however. For example, the Craniosacral Therapy Association (CSTA) registers craniosacral practitioners in the UK. This includes biodynamic practitioners, but its members are not necessarily biodynamic practitioners. Some other countries, like Italy and Spain, have biodynamic associations.

The information here is by no means all-inclusive. It is not possible to list all schools in the world offering biodynamic training. I have limited this list to trainings developed or offered by Franklyn Sills. Please refer to the associations listed for specific schools in your region. Unfortunately, you may not find schools in your area, but that is gradually changing, with Craniosacral Biodynamics spreading to hungry practitioners around the world.

I hope this book and these resources support you in feeding whatever urges you may have to pursue or understand more deeply this beautiful work.

May you know the ever-present support of the Breath of Life as you walk your path, wherever it may lead.

NOTES

1   L. N. Vandenberg, R. D. Morrie, and D. S. Adams, "V-ATPase-Dependent Ectodermal Voltage and pH Regionalization Are Required for Craniofacial Morphogenesis," *Developmental Dynamics* 240 (2011): 1889–1904.

2   Bonnie Gintis, *Engaging the Movement of Life: Exploring Health and Embodiment Through Osteopathy and Continuum* (Berkeley, CA: North Atlantic Books, 2007), 79.

3   Franklyn Sills, *Foundations in Craniosacral Biodynamics: The Breath of Life and Fundamental Skills, Vol. 1* (Berkeley, CA: North Atlantic Books, 2011), 207.

4   Rollin E. Becker, *Life in Motion: The Osteopathic View of Rollin E. Becker* (Portland, OR: Stillness Press, 1997), 157.

5   Erich Blechschmidt and R. F. Gasser, *Biokinetics and Biodynamics of Human Differentiation: Principles and Applications* (Springfield, IL: Charles C. Thomas, 1978).

6   Oxford English Living Dictionary, s.v. "morphology," https://en.oxforddictionaries.com/definition/morphology.

7   John Upledger, *Your Inner Physician and You* (Berkeley, CA: North Atlantic Books, 1991).

8   Andrew Taylor Still, *Philosophy and Mechanical Principles of Osteopathy* (Kirksville, MO: Osteopathic Enterprises, 1986), 44–45.

9   William Garner Sutherland, ed. A. L. Wales, *Teachings in the Science of Osteopathy* (Fort Worth, TX: Sutherland Cranial Teaching Foundation, 1990), 3–4.

10 Adah Strand Sutherland, *With Thinking Fingers: The Story of William Garner Sutherland* (Indianapolis, IN: The Cranial Academy, 1962), 34.

11 Sills, *Foundations in Craniosacral Biodynamics*, 7.

12 William Garner Sutherland, *The Cranial Bowl: A Treatise Relating to Cranial Articular Mobility, Cranial Articular Lesions and Cranial Technic* (Berkeley, CA: The Free Press, 1978), 3.

13 William Garner Sutherland, *Contributions of Thought: The Collected Writings of William Garner Sutherland, D.O.,* ed. A. D. Sutherland and A. L. Wales (Fort Worth, TX: Sutherland Cranial Teaching Foundation, 1998).

14 Sutherland, *Teachings in the Science of Osteopathy*.

15 Becker, *Life in Motion*.

16 Ibid., 203.

17 Ho, Mae-Wan, *The Rainbow and the Worm: The Physics of Organisms,* 3rd ed. (London: World Scientific Publishing, 2008).

18 Tufts University, "The Face of a Frog." YouTube video posted July 22, 2011, https://www.youtube.com/watch?v=ndFe5CaDTlI.

19 Sills, *Foundations in Craniosacral Biodynamics.*

20 Sarah Knapton, "Bright Flash of Light Marks Incredible Moment Life Begins When Sperm Meets Egg," *The Telegraph,* April 26, 2016, http://www.telegraph.co.uk/science/2016/04/26/bright-flash-of-light-marks-incredible-moment-life-begins-when-s.

21 Sutherland, *Contributions of Thought.*

22 Andrew Taylor Still, *Philosophy of Osteopathy* (Kirksville, MO: A.T. Still, 1899), 28.

23 Becker, *Life in Motion,* 157.

24 Sutherland, *Contributions of Thought,* 14.

25 Becker, *Life in Motion.*

26 Sutherland, as cited in Becker, *Life in Motion.*

27 Franklyn Sills, personal communication.

28 Sills, *Foundations in Craniosacral Biodynamics.*

29 Begley as cited in Bonnie Badenoch, *Being a Brain-Wise Therapist: A Practical Guide to Interpersonal Neurobiology* (New York: W. W. Norton, 2008).

30 e.g., Masaru Emoto, *The Hidden Messages in Water,* trans. David A. Thayne (Hillsboro, OR: Beyond Words Publishing, 2004); and William A. Tiller, Walter E. Dibble, Jr., and Michael J. Kohane, *Conscious Acts of Creation: The Emergence of a New Physics* (Walnut Creek, CA: Pavior, 2001).

31 Anna Chitty, personal communication, Boulder, CO, 2003.

32 David Bohm, *Wholeness and the Implicate Order* (London: Routledge, 1980), 13.

33 Bruce Lipton, "New Biology Healthcare Revolution: Genes Do Not Control Biology," *World Summit of Integrative Medicine,* 2015, http://worldsummitintegrativemedicine.com/dr-bruce-lipton/.

34 Karel Schrijver and Iris Schrijver, *Living with the Stars: How the Human Body Is Connected to the Life Cycles of the Earth, the Planets, and the Stars* (Oxford: Oxford University Press, 2015).

35 Donald W. Winnicott, *The Maturational Processes and the Facilitating Environment: Studies in the Theory of Emotional Development,* rev. ed. (London: Karnac, 2007).

36 Ibid., 47.

37   e.g., Daniel J. Siegel, *The Mindful Brain: Reflection and Attunement in the Cultivation of Well-Being* (New York: W. W. Norton, 2007).

38   Tara Brach, "The Reality of Change: Embracing This Living Dying World" (podcast) May 24, 2017, https://www.tarabrach.com/reality-change/.

39   Stephen W. Porges, "The Polyvagal Theory: Phylogenetic Substrates of a Social Nervous System," *International Journal of Psychophysiology* 42 (2001): 123–46.

40   Ravi Dykema, "How Your Nervous System Sabotages Your Ability to Relate: An Interview with Stephen Porges about His Polyvagal Theory." *Nexus: Colorado's Holistic Health and Spirituality Journal* (March/April, 2006), https://nexusalive.com/articles/interviews/stephen-porges-ph-d-the-polyvagel-theory/.

41   Rollin McCraty, *The Energetic Heart: Biomechanic Interactions Within and Between People* (Boulder Creek, CA: HeartMath Institute, 2003), 1.

42   Frédérick Leboyer, *Birth without Violence* (New York: Alfred A. Knopf, 1975).

43   Dykema, "How Your Nervous System Sabotages Your Ability to Relate."

44   Sills, *Foundations in Craniosacral Biodynamics.*

45   Sills. *Being and Becoming,* 4.

46   Winnicott, *The Maturational Processes and the Facilitating Environment,* 47.

47   Tara Brach, "Interview with Tami Simon," *Insights from the Edge* (podcast), August 13, 2013. http://www.soundstrue.com/podcast/transcripts/tara-brach.php?camefromhome=camefromhome.

48   Laura Dethiville. *Donald W. Winnicott: A New Approach,* trans. Susan Ganley Lévy. (London: Karnac, 2014), 6.

49   Winnicott, *The Maturational Processes and the Facilitating Environment.*

50   e.g., Carl R. Rogers, "The Necessary and Sufficient Conditions of Therapeutic Personality Change," *Journal of Consulting Psychology* 21 (1957): 95–103; and Young, 2010.

51   e.g., Dykema, "How Your Nervous System Sabotages Your Ability to Relate."

52   Rollin McCraty and Doc Childre, *The Intuitive Heart: Accessing Inner Guidance to Raise Our Consciousness Baseline* (Boulder Creek, CA: HeartMath Institute, 2014), 12.

53   Diane Poole Heller and Laurence S. Heller, *Crash Course. A Self-Healing Guide to Auto Accident Trauma and Recovery* (Berkeley, CA: North Atlantic, 2001), xx.

54   Personal communication, Franklyn Sills, November 26, 2014.

55   Winnicott, *The Maturational Processes and the Facilitating Environment.*

56 Margin Buber, *I and Thou,* 2nd ed., trans. Ronald Gregor Smith (New York: Scribner's, 1958), 28.

57 e.g., R. Block and N. F. Krebs, "Failure to Thrive as a Manifestation of Child Neglect." *Pediatrics* 116, no. 5 (2005): 1234–37.

58 e.g., Lipton, 2005.

59 e.g., Peter W. Nathanielsz, *Life in the Womb: The Origin of Health and Disease* (n.p.: Promethean Press, 1999).

60 Gabor Maté, *Scattered: How Attention Deficit Disorder Originates and What You Can Do About It* (London: Plume, 2000), 43.

61 Donald W. Winnicott, *Playing and Reality* (London: Penguin, 1971), 103.

62 Winnicott, *The Maturational Processes and the Facilitating Environment.*

63 Franklyn Sills, *Foundations in Craniosacral Biodynamics: The Sentient Embryo, Tissue Intelligence, and Trauma Resolution, Vol. 2.* (Berkeley, CA: North Atlantic Books, 2012).

64 Donald W. Winnicott, *Playing and Reality.*

65 Lynne McTaggart, *The Field: The Quest for the Secret Force of the Universe,* updated ed. (New York: Harper, 2001), 66–67.

66 Ibid.

67 Lynne McTaggart, *The Intention Experiment: Use Your Thoughts to Change the World* (New York, Harper Element, 2008); and Lynne McTaggart, *The Power of Eight: Harnessing the Miraculous Energies of a Small Group to Heal Others, Your Life, and the World* (New York: Atria, 2017).

68 James L. Oschman, *Energy Medicine: The Scientific Basis* (Edinburgh: Churchill Livingstone, 2000).

69 Rollin McCraty and Annette Deyhle, *The Science of Interconnectivity: Exploring the Human-Earth Connection* (Boulder Creek, CA: HeartMath Institute, 2016).

70 e.g., Masaru Emoto, presentation at the University of California, Santa Barbara, May 18, 2005.

71 Ibid.

72 Masaru Emoto, *The Hidden Messages in Water* (New York: Pocket, 2005).

73 William A. Tiller, Walter E. Dibble, Jr., and Michael J. Kohane, *Conscious Acts of Creation: The Emergence of a New Physics* (Walnut Creek, CA: Pavior, 2001).

74 William A. Tiller, and Cynthia R. Reed. "White Paper XVI: The Effect of Intention on Decreasing Human Depression and Anxiety Via Broadcasting from an Intention-Host Device-Conditioned Experimental Space," 2005, www.tiller.org.

75 Emilie Conrad, "The Art of Self Renewal: The Fluid System," *Continuum Movement,* accessed December 16, 2015, http://www.continuummovement.com/ov-fluid.php.

76 Genesis 2:7 (King James Bible).

77 Genesis 2:6 (King James Bible).

78 Still, *Philosophy and Mechanical Principles of Osteopathy,* 44–45.

79 Sutherland, *With Thinking Fingers,* 13.

80 e.g., Sutherland, *Contributions of Thought.*

81 Still, *Philosophy and Mechanical Principles of Osteopathy,* 44–45.

82 Sutherland, *Contributions of Thought,* 142.

83 Sutherland, *Teachings in the Science of Osteopathy,* 14.

84 Michael Kern, *Wisdom in the Body: The Craniosacral Approach to Essential Health* (Berkeley, CA: North Atlantic, 2005), 138.

85 e.g., Malcolm Hiort "C.R.I. Rates: A Critical Review of the Literature Reporting the Rate of the Cranial Rhythmic Impulse," research project at Victoria University of Technology, 1997, http://craniofascial.com/post-number-1/; and Nicette Sergueef, Melissa A. Greer, Kenneth E. Nelson, and Thomas Glonek. "The Palpated Cranial Rhythmic Impulse (CRI): Its Normative Rate and Examiner Experience," *International Journal of Osteopathic Medicine* 14, no. 1 (March 2011): 10–16.

86 Sills, *Foundations in Craniosacral Biodynamics,* 119.

87 Ibid., 145.

88 Rollin E. Becker, *The Stillness of Life: The Osteopathic Philosophy of Rollin E. Becker* (Portland, OR: Stillness Press, 2000), 49–50.

89 William Seifritz, "Protoplasm of a Slime Mold: The Stuff of Life." 1954. Published on You Tube as "Seifritz on Protoplasm—Full Film," June 24, 2015. https://youtu.be/_ihSxAn4WR8.

90 e.g., Vince Stricherz, "Listening to the Big Bang—In High Fidelity (audio)," University of Washington: UW Today, April 4, 2013, http://www.washington.edu/news/2013/04/04/listening-to-the-big-bang-in-high-fidelity-audio/.

91 Sills, *Foundations in Craniosacral Biodynamics,* 17.

92 Becker, *The Stillness of Life,* 30.

93 Ibid., 30.

94 Ibid, 30–31.

95 Bohm, *Wholeness and the Implicate Order,* xv.

96 Hongzhi, *Cultivating the Empty Field: The Silent Illumination of Zen Master Hongzhi,* trans. Taigen Daniel Leighton (San Francisco: North Point, 1991), 5.

97 Psalm 46:10 (King James Bible).

98 Becker, *The Stillness of Life*, 122.

99 Sills, *Foundations in Craniosacral Biodynamics*, 311.

100 Ho, *The Rainbow and the Worm*, 2008.

101 Sills, *Foundations in Craniosacral Biodynamics*, 292.

102 Mary Oliver, "The Messenger," *Thirst: Poems* (Boston: Beacon, 2006).

103 Becker, *The Stillness of Life*, 46.

104 Ibid, 43.

105 Sills, *Foundations in Craniosacral Biodynamics*, 51.

106 Becker, *Life in Motion.*

107 Thich Nhat Hanh, *Peace Is Every Step: The Path of Mindfulness in Everyday Life* (New York: Bantam Books, 1991), 77.

108 Online Etymology Dictionary, accessed July 1, 2017, http://www.etymonline.com/.

109 Still, *Philosophy of Osteopathy*, 28.

110 Becker, *Life in Motion*, 125.

111 Ibid., 157.

112 Franklyn Sills, *The Three Functions of Potency* (unpublished manuscript), 2015.

113 Lizzie Velasquez, "How Do YOU Define Yourself at TEDxAustinWomen," published on YouTube December 20, 2013, https://youtu.be/c62Aqdlzvqk.

114 Becker, *Life in Motion*, 183.

115 Sills, *Foundations in Craniosacral Biodynamics*, 52.

116 Jon Kabat-Zinn, *Full Catastrophe Living* (New York: Delta, 1990), 161.

117 Seifritz, "Protoplasm of a Slime Mold."

118 Becker, *The Stillness of Life*, 113.

119 Franklyn Sills, *Foundations in Craniosacral Biodynamics*, rev. ed. (Berkeley, CA: North Atlantic, 2016).

120 Sills, *Foundations in Craniosacral Biodynamics*, 53.

121 Ibid.

122 Rollin McCraty and Doc Childre, "Coherence: Bridging Personal, Social and Global Health," *Alternative Therapies in Health and Medicine* 14, no. 4 (2010): 10–24.

123 Sills, *Foundations in Craniosacral Biodynamics*, 214.

124 Ibid., 226.

125 Becker, *Life in Motion.*

126 Sills, *Foundations in Craniosacral Biodynamics*, 234.

127 Becker, *Life in Motion*, 182.

128 Ibid.

129 Knapton, "Bright Flash of Light Marks Incredible Moment."

130 Francesca E. Duncan, Emily L. Que, Nan Zhang, Eve C. Feinberg, Thomas V. O'Halloran, and Teresa K. Woodruff. "The Zinc Spark Is an Inorganic Signature of Human Egg Activation," *Scientific Reports* 6, published electronically April 26, 2016, doi: 10.1038/srep24737.

131 Franklyn Sills, *Foundations in Craniosacral Biodynamics*, 226.

132 Alick Bartholomew, *Hidden Nature: The Startling Insights of Viktor Schauberger* (Edinburgh: Floris, 2003), 66.

133 Ibid., 60.

134 Ibid., 27.

135 Arthur T. Winfree, *When Time Breaks Down: The Three-Dimensional Dynamics of Electrochemical Waves and Cardiac Arrhythmias* (Princeton: Princeton University Press, 1987).

136 Vandenberg, Morrie, and Adams, "V-ATPase-Dependent Ectodermal Voltage and pH Regionalization."

137 Jaap Van der Wal and Guus van der Bie, "The Incarnating Embryo—The Embryo in Us: Human Embryonic Development in a Phenomenological Perspective," chap. 10 in *Osteopathic Energetics: Morphodynamic and Biodynamic Principles in Health and Disease,* ed. Torsten Liem (Pencaitland, Scotland: Handspring, 2016).

138 Emilie Conrad, *Life on Land: The Story of Continuum, the World-Renowned Self-Discovery and Movement Method* (Berkeley, CA: North Atlantic, 2007).

139 Erich Blechschmidt and R. F. Gasser, *The Ontogenetic Basis of Human Anatomy: A Biodynamic Approach to Development from Conception to Birth* (Berkeley, CA: North Atlantic, 2004), 61.

140 Bruce Lipton, *The Biology of Belief: Unleashing the Power of Consciousness, Matter, and Miracles* (Carlsbad, CA: Hay House, 2005).

141 Blechschmidt and Gasser, *The Ontogenetic Basis of Human Anatomy*, 61.

142 William Emerson, personal communication, July 1994.

143 Sills, *Foundations in Craniosacral Biodynamic*, 300.

144 Peter Levine, *Waking the Tiger: Healing Trauma* (Berkeley, CA: North Atlantic, 1997), 12.

145 e.g., Bessel Van Der Kolk, *The Body Keeps the Score: Mind, Brain and Body in the Transformation of Trauma* (New York: Penguin, 2015); Peter Levine, *Waking the Tiger*; Peter Levine, *In an Unspoken Voice: How the Body Releases Trauma and Restores Goodness* (Berkeley, CA; North Atlantic, 2010); Peter Levine, *Trauma and Memory: Brain and Body in Search of the Living Past: A Practical Guide for Understanding and Working with Traumatic Memory* (Berkeley, CA: North Atlantic, 2015); and Gabor Maté, *When the Body Says No: The Cost of Hidden Stress* (Toronto: Random House, 2012).

146 e.g., Maté, *When the Body Says No*; and Sills, *Foundations in Craniosacral Biodynamics Vol. 2.*

147 Ruth Buczynski, "Recognizing the Risk of PTSD in Our Patients, *NICABM,* accessed June 17, 2015, https://www.nicabm.com/nicabmblog/recognizing-risk-ptsd-patients/.

148 Peter Levine, "Memory, Trauma, and Healing," *International Trauma-Healing Institute,* accessed August 24, 2016, http://healingtrauma.org.il/resources/articles/memory-trauma-healing.

149 Sandor Szabo, "The Creative and Productive Life of Hans Selye: A Review of His Major Scientific Discoveries," *Experientia* 4, no. 5 (1985): 564.

150 Blechschmidt and Gasser, *Biokinetics and Biodynamics of Human Differentiation.*

151 Blechschmidt and Glasser, *The Ontogenetic Basis of Human Anatomy.*

152 Van der Wal and van der Bie. "The Incarnating Embryo."

153 Sarah J. Buckley, *Gentle Birth, Gentle Mothering: A Doctor's Guide to Natural Childbirth and Gentle Early Parenting Choices* (Berkeley, CA: Celestial Arts, 2009).

154 Jean Liedloff, *The Continuum Concept: Allowing Human Nature to Work Successfully* (New York: Addison-Wesley, 1994).

155 Ibid., 24

156 Ibid., 26.

157 C. Beck, referenced by Penny Simpkin, *The Significance of Childbirth to the Birthing Person: Influences of Care and Place for Birth* (webinar) 2015, https://www.goldlearning.com/lecture-library/live-webinar/significance-of-childbirth-public-detail.

158 David Chamberlain, "What Babies Are Teaching Us About Violence," *Journal of Prenatal and Perinatal Psychology and Health* 10, no. 2 (1995): 51–74.

159 David Chamberlain, *The Mind of Your Newborn Baby* (Berkeley, CA: North Atlantic, 1998).

160 Thomas Verny and John Kelly, *The Secret Life of the Unborn Child* (New York: Delta, 1981).

161 e.g., Porges, "The Polyvagal Theory," 123–46; and Stephen Porges, *The Polyvagal Theory: Neurophysiological Foundations of Emotions, Attachment, Communication, and Self-Regulation* (New York: W. W. Norton, 2011).

162 e.g., Vincent J. Felitti, Robert F. Anda, Dale Nordenberg, David F. Williamson, Alison M. Spitz, Valerie Edwards, Mary P. Koss, and James S. Marks, "Relationship of Childhood Abuse and Household Dysfunction to Many of the Leading Causes of Death in Adults," *American Journal of Preventive Medicine* 14, no. 4 (1998): 245–58; and Vincent J. Felitti, "Adverse Childhood Experiences and Adult Health," *Academic Pediatrics* 9 (2009): 131–32.

163 Dykema, "How Your Nervous System Sabotages Your Ability to Relate."

164 Steven W. Porges and Ruth Buczynski, "The Polyvagal Theory for Treating Trauma," accessed June 17, 2015, http://stephenporges.com/images/stephen%20porges%20interview%20nicabm.pdf, 11.

165 Ibid.

166 Ibid.

167 Levine, "Memory, Trauma, and Healing."

168 Porges and Buczynski, "The Polyvagal Theory for Treating Trauma."

169 Becker, *Life in Motion*, 125.

170 Levine, *Waking the Tiger*.

171 e.g., Siegel, *The Mindful Brain*; and Daniel J. Siegel, "Mindfulness Training and Neural Integration: Differentiation of Distinct Streams of Awareness and the Cultivation of Well-Being," *Social Cognitive and Affective Neuroscience* 2, no. 4 (2007): 259–63.

172 Christine Caldwell, *Getting Our Bodies Back: Recovery, Healing and Transformation Through Body-Centered Psychotherapy* (Boston: Shambala, 1996).

173 e.g., Antonio Damasio, *Self Comes to Mind: Constructing the Conscious Brain* (New York: Vintage, 2012).

174 e.g., Stephen W. Porges, "The Polyvagal Perspective," *Biological Psychology* 74, no. 2 (2007): 116–43.

175 Becker, *The Stillness of Life*, 243.

176 Sills, *Foundations in Craniosacral Biodynamics*, 357.

177 Becker, *The Stillness of Life*, 32.

178 Lisa Kalinowska and Daska Hatton, *Every Body Tells a Story: A Craniosacral Journey* (London: Singing Dragon, 2016), 10.

REFERENCES

American Psychiatric Association. *Diagnostic and Statistical Manual of Mental Disorders.* 5th ed. Washington, D.C.: American Psychiatric Association, 2013.

Badenoch, Bonnie. *Being a Brain-Wise Therapist: A Practical Guide to Interpersonal Neurobiology.* New York: W. W. Norton, 2008.

Bartholomew, Alick. *Hidden Nature: The Startling Insights of Viktor Schauberger.* Edinburgh: Floris, 2003.

Becker, Rollin E. *Life in Motion: The Osteopathic View of Rollin E. Becker.* Portland, OR: Stillness Press, 1997.

———. *The Stillness of Life: The Osteopathic Philosophy of Rollin E. Becker.* Portland, OR: Stillness Press, 2000.

Blechschmidt, Erich, and R. F. Gasser. *Biokinetics and Biodynamics of Human Differentiation: Principles and Applications.* Springfield, IL: Charles C. Thomas, 1978.

———. *The Ontogenetic Basis of Human Anatomy: A Biodynamic Approach to Development from Conception to Birth.* Berkeley, CA: North Atlantic, 2004.

Block, R., and N. F. Krebs. "Failure to Thrive as a Manifestation of Child Neglect." *Pediatrics* 116, no. 5 (2005): 1234–37.

Bohm, David. *Wholeness and the Implicate Order.* London: Routledge, 1980.

Brach, Tara. "Interview with Tami Simon." *Insights from the Edge* (podcast). August 13, 2013. http://www.soundstrue.com/podcast/transcripts/tara-brach.php?camefrom home=camefromhome.

———. *The Reality of Change: Embracing This Living Dying World* (podcast). May 24, 2017. https://www.tarabrach.com/reality-change/.

Buber, Martin. *I and Thou,* 2nd ed. Translated by Ronald Gregor Smith. New York: Scribner's, 1958.

Buckley, Sarah J. *Gentle Birth, Gentle Mothering: A Doctor's Guide to Natural Childbirth and Gentle Early Parenting Choices.* Berkeley, CA: Celestial Arts, 2009.

Buczynski, Ruth. "Recognizing the Risk of PTSD in Our Patients." *NICABM*. Accessed June 17, 2015. https://www.nicabm.com/nicabmblog/recognizing-risk-ptsd-patients/.

Caldwell, Christine. *Getting Our Bodies Back: Recovery, Healing and Transformation Through Body-Centered Psychotherapy.* Boston: Shambala, 1996.

Chamberlain, David. "What Babies Are Teaching Us about Violence." *Journal of Prenatal and Perinatal Psychology and Health* 10, no. 2 (1995): 51–74.

———. *The Mind of Your Newborn Baby.* Berkeley, CA: North Atlantic, 1998.

Conrad, Emilie. *Life on Land: The Story of Continuum, the World-Renowned Self-Discovery and Movement Method.* Berkeley, CA: North Atlantic, 2007.

———. "The Art of Self Renewal: The Fluid System." *Continuum Movement.* Accessed December 16, 2015. http://continuummovement.com/the-art-of-self-renewal-the-fluid-system/.

Damasio, Antonio. *Self Comes to Mind: Constructing the Conscious Brain.* New York: Vintage, 2012.

Dethiville, Laura. *Donald W. Winnicott: A New Approach.* Translated by Susan Ganley Lévy. London: Karnac, 2014.

Duncan, Francesca E., Emily L. Que, Nan Zhang, Eve C. Feinberg, Thomas V. O'Halloran, and Teresa K. Woodruff. "The Zinc Spark Is an Inorganic Signature of Human Egg Activation." *Scientific Reports* 6. Published electronically April 26, 2016. doi: 10.1038/srep24737.

Dykema, Ravi. "How Your Nervous System Sabotages Your Ability to Relate: An Interview with Stephen Porges about His Polyvagal Theory." *Nexus: Colorado's Holistic Health and Spirituality Journal* (March/April, 2006). https://nexusalive.com/articles/interviews/stephen-porges-ph-d-the-polyvagal-theory.

Emoto, Masaru. *The Hidden Messages in Water.* Translated by David A. Thayne. Hillsboro, OR: Beyond Words Publishing, 2004.

———. *The Hidden Messages in Water.* New York: Pocket, 2005.

———. Presentation at the University of California, Santa Barbara, May 18, 2005.

Felitti, Vincent J. "Adverse Childhood Experiences and Adult Health." *Academic Pediatrics* 9 (2009): 131–32.

Felitti, Vincent J., Robert F. Anda, Dale Nordenberg, David F. Williamson, Alison M. Spitz, Valerie Edwards, Mary P. Koss, and James S. Marks. "Relationship of Childhood Abuse and Household Dysfunction to Many of the Leading Causes of Death in Adults." *American Journal of Preventive Medicine* 14, no. 4 (1998): 245–58.

Gintis, Bonnie. *Engaging the Movement of Life: Exploring Health and Embodiment Through Osteopathy and Continuum.* Berkeley, CA: North Atlantic, 2007.

Grey, Alex. *Transfigurations.* Rochester, VT: Inner Traditions, 2001.

Heller, Diane Poole, and Laurence S. Heller. *Crash Course: A Self-Healing Guide to Auto Accident Trauma and Recovery.* Berkeley, CA: North Atlantic, 2001

Hiort, Malcolm. "C.R.I. Rates: A Critical Review of the Literature Reporting the Rate of the Cranial Rhythmic Impulse." Research project at Victoria University of Technology, 1997. http://craniofascial.com/post-number-1/.

Ho, Mae-Wan. *The Rainbow and the Worm: The Physics of Organisms,* 3rd ed. London: World Scientific Publishing, 2008.

Hongzhi. *Cultivating the Empty Field: The Silent Illumination of Zen Master Hongzhi.* Translated by Taigen Daniel Leighton. New York: North Point, 1991.

Kabat-Zinn, Jon. *Full Catastrophe Living.* New York: Delta, 1990.

Kalinowska, Liz, and Daska Hatton. *Every Body Tells a Story: A Craniosacral Journey.* London: Singing Dragon, 2016

Kern, Michael. *Wisdom in the Body: The Craniosacral Approach to Essential Health.* Berkeley, CA: North Atlantic, 2005.

Knapton, Sarah. "Bright Flash of Light Marks Incredible Moment Life Begins When Sperm Meets Egg." *The Telegraph,* April 26, 2016. http://www.telegraph.co.uk/science/2016/04/26/bright-flash-of-light-marks-incredible-moment-life-begins-when-s.

Leboyer, Frédérick. *Birth without Violence.* New York: Alfred A. Knopf, 1975.

Levine, Peter. *In an Unspoken Voice: How the Body Releases Trauma and Restores Goodness.* Berkeley, CA: North Atlantic, 2010.

———. "Memory, Trauma, and Healing." *International Trauma-Healing Institute.* Accessed August 24, 2016. http://healingtrauma.org.il/resources/articles/memory-trauma-healing.

————. *Trauma and Memory: Brain and Body in Search of the Living Past: A Practical Guide for Understanding and Working with Traumatic Memory.* Berkeley, CA: North Atlantic, 2015.

————. *Waking the Tiger: Healing Trauma.* Berkeley, CA: North Atlantic, 1997.

Liedloff, Jean. *The Continuum Concept: Allowing Human Nature to Work Successfully.* New York: Addison-Wesley, 1977.

Lipton, Bruce. *Biology of Belief: Unleashing the Power of Consciousness, Matter, and Miracles.* Carlsbad, CA: Hay House, 2008.

————. "New Biology Healthcare Revolution: Genes Do Not Control Biology." *World Summit of Integrative Medicine.* 2015. http://worldsummitintegrativemedicine .com/dr-bruce-lipton.

Maté, Gabor. *Scattered: How Attention Deficit Disorder Originates and What You Can Do About It.* London: Plume, 2000.

————. *When the Body Says No: The Cost of Hidden Stress.* Toronto: Random House, 2012.

McCraty, Rollin. *The Energetic Heart: Bioelectromagnetic Communication Within and Between People.* Boulder Creek, CA: HeartMath Institute, 2003.

McCraty Rollin, and Doc Childre. "Coherence: Bridging Personal, Social and Global Health." *Alternative Therapies in Health and Medicine* 14, no. 4 (2010): 10–24.

————. *The Intuitive Heart: Accessing Inner Guidance to Raise Our Consciousness Baseline.* Boulder Creek, CA: HeartMath Institute, 2014.

McCraty, Rollin, and Annette Deyhle. *The Science of Interconnectivity: Exploring the Human-Earth Connection.* Boulder Creek, CA: HeartMath Institute, 2016.

McTaggart, Lynne. *The Bond: The Power of Connection.* Carlsbad, CA: Hay House, 2013.

————. *The Field: The Quest for the Secret Force of the Universe.* Updated ed. New York: Harper, 2001.

————. *The Intention Experiment: Use Your Thoughts to Change the World.* New York: Harper Element, 2008.

————. *The Power of Eight: Harnessing the Miraculous Energies of a Small Group to Heal Others, Your Life, and the World.* New York: Atria, 2017.

Nathanielsz, Peter W. *Life in the Womb: The Origin of Health and Disease.* n.p.: Promethean Press, 1999.

Oliver, Mary. "The Messenger." *Thirst: Poems.* Boston: Beacon, 2006.

Oschman, James L. *Energy Medicine: The Scientific Basis.* Edinburgh: Churchill Livingstone, 2000.

Porges, Stephen W. *The Polyvagal Theory: Neurophysiological Foundations of Emotions, Attachment, Communication, and Self-Regulation.* New York: W. W. Norton, 2011.

———. "The Polyvagal Theory: Phylogenetic Substrates of a Social Nervous System." *International Journal of Psychophysiology* 42 (2001): 123–46.

———. "The Polyvagal Perspective." *Biological Psychology* 74, no. 2 (2007): 116–43.

Porges, Stephen W., and Ruth Buczynski, "The Polyvagal Theory for Treating Trauma." Accessed June 17, 2015. http://stephenporges.com/images/stephen%20porges%20interview%20nicabm.pdf.

Rogers, Carl R. "The Necessary and Sufficient Conditions of Therapeutic Personality Change." *Journal of Consulting Psychology* 21 (1957): 95–103.

Sadler, T. W. (2010). *Langman's Medical Embryology.* 11th ed. International ed. London: Lippincott Williams and Wilkins, 2010.

Schoenwolf, Gary C., Steven B. Bleyl, Philip R. Brauer, and Philippa H. Francis-West. *Larsen's Hyman Embryology,* 4th ed. Edinburgh: Churchill Livingstone, 2009.

Schrijver, Karel, and Iris Schrijver. *Living with the Stars: How the Human Body Is Connected to the Life Cycles of the Earth, the Planets, and the Stars.* Oxford: Oxford University Press, 2015.

Seifritz, William. "Protoplasm of a Slime Mold: The Stuff of Life." 1954. Published on You Tube as "Seifritz on Protoplasm—Full Film," June 24, 2015. https://youtu.be/_ihSxAn4WR8.

Sergueef, Nicette, Melissa A. Greer, Kenneth E. Nelson, and Thomas Glonek. "The Palpated Cranial Rhythmic Impulse (CRI): Its Normative Rate and Examiner Experience." *International Journal of Osteopathic Medicine* 14, no. 1 (March 2011): 10–16.

Siegel, Daniel J. *The Mindful Brain: Reflection and Attunement in the Cultivation of Well-Being.* New York: W. W. Norton, 2007.

————. "Mindfulness Training and Neural Integration: Differentiation of Distinct Streams of Awareness and the Cultivation of Well-Being." *Social Cognitive and Affective Neuroscience* 2, no. 4 (2007): 259–63.

Sills, Franklyn. *Being and Becoming: Psychodynamics, Buddhism, and the Origins of Selfhood*. Berkeley, CA: North Atlantic, 2008.

————. *Craniosacral Biodynamics, Vol 1: The Breath of Life, Biodynamics, and Foundational Skills*. Berkeley, CA: North Atlantic, 2001.

————. *Foundations in Craniosacral Biodynamics: The Breath of Life and Fundamental Skills, Vol. 1*. Berkeley, CA: North Atlantic Books, 2011.

————. *Foundations in Craniosacral Biodynamics: The Sentient Embryo, Tissue Intelligence, and Trauma Resolution, Vol. 2*. Berkeley, CA: North Atlantic Books, 2012.

————. *Foundations in Craniosacral Biodynamics*. Revised ed. Berkeley, CA: North Atlantic, 2016.

————. "The Relational Field and Empathy." *Craniosacral Biodynamics*. 2012. Accessed November 26, 2014. http://www.craniosacral-biodynamics.org/articles-relational-field-empathy.html.

————. "The Three Functions of Potency." Unpublished manuscript. 2015.

Simpkin, Penny. *The Significance of Childbirth to the Birthing Person: Influences of Care and Place for Birth*. Webinar filmed 2015. https://www.goldlearning.com/lecture-library/live-webinar/significance-of-childbirth-public-detail.

Still, Andrew Taylor. *Philosophy of Osteopathy*. Kirksville, MO: A.T. Still, 1899.

————. *Philosophy and Mechanical Principles of Osteopathy*. Kirksville, MO: Osteopathic Enterprises, 1986.

Stricherz, Vince. "Listening to the Big Bang—In High Fidelity (audio)." University of Washington: UW Today. April 4, 2013. http://www.washington.edu/news/2013/04/04/listening-to-the-big-bang-in-high-fidelity-audio/.

Sutherland, Adah Strand. *With Thinking Fingers: The Story of William Garner Sutherland*. Indianapolis, IN: The Cranial Academy, 1962.

Sutherland, William Garner. *Contributions of Thought: The Collected Writings of William Garner Sutherland, D.O.* Edited by A. D. Sutherland and A. L. Wales. Fort Worth, TX: Sutherland Cranial Teaching Foundation, 1998.

———. *The Cranial Bowl: A Treatise Relating to Cranial Articular Mobility, Cranial Articular Lesions, and Cranial Technic.* Berkeley, CA: The Free Press, 1978.

———. *Teachings in the Science of Osteopathy.* Edited by A. L. Wales. Fort Worth, TX: Sutherland Cranial Teaching Foundation, 1990.

Szabo, Sandor. "The Creative and Productive Life of Hans Selye: A Review of His Major Scientific Discoveries." *Experientia* 4, no. 5 (1985): 564–67.

Thich Nhat Hanh. *Peace Is Every Step: The Path of Mindfulness in Everyday Life.* New York: Bantam Books, 1991.

Tiller, William A., Walter E. Dibble, Jr., and Michael J. Kohane, *Conscious Acts of Creation: The Emergence of a New Physics.* Walnut Creek, CA: Pavior, 2001.

Tiller, William A., and Cynthia R. Reed. "White Paper XVI: The Effect of Intention on Decreasing Human Depression and Anxiety Via Broadcasting from an Intention-Host Device-Conditioned Experimental Space." 2005. www.tiller.org.

Tufts University. "The Face of a Frog." Published on YouTube July 22, 2011. https://www.youtube.com/watch?v=ndFe5CaDTlI.

Upledger, John. *Your Inner Physician and You: Craniosacral Therapy and Somatoemotional Release.* Berkeley, CA: North Atlantic, 1991.

Vandenberg, L. N., R. D. Morrie, and D. S. Adams. "V-ATPase-Dependent Ectodermal Voltage and pH Regionalization Are Required for Craniofacial Morphogenesis." *Developmental Dynamics* 240 (2011): 1889–1904.

Van der Kolk, Bessel. *The Body Keeps the Score: Mind, Brain and Body in the Transformation of Trauma.* New York: Penguin, 2015.

Van der Wal, Jaap, and Guus van der Bie. "The Incarnating Embryo—The Embryo in Us: Human Embryonic Development in a Phenomenological Perspective." Chap. 10 in *Osteopathic Energetics: Morphodynamic and Biodynamic Principles in Health and Disease,* edited by Torsten Liem. Pencaitland, Scotland: Handspring, 2016.

Velasquez, Lizzie. "How Do YOU Define Yourself at TEDxAustinWomen." Published on YouTube December 20, 2013. https://youtu.be/c62Aqdlzvqk.

Verny, Thomas, and John Kelly. *The Secret Life of the Unborn Child.* New York: Delta, 1981.

Winfree, Arthur T. *When Time Breaks Down: The Three-Dimensional Dynamics of Electrochemical Waves and Cardiac Arrhythmias.* Princeton: Princeton University Press, 1987.

Winnicott, Donald W. *The Maturational Processes and the Facilitating Environment: Studies in the Theory of Emotional Development.* Revised ed. London: Karnac, 2007.

———. *Playing and Reality.* London: Penguin, 1971.

INDEX

settling defensive neural patterning, 55–56
shifting out of defensive states, 50
space, contact, and respect and, 57
Western world under influence of over-active
    sympathetic nervous systems, 27–29

T

temporomandibular joint (TMJ), 191
tensegrity (Fuller), 76
Thich Nhat Hanh, 98, 199
"Three Body Chi Kung," 17, 188
The Three Functions of Potency, and Brain, and
    Heart and Being seminar, 198
tidal waves
    cranial. *see* cranial rhythmic impulse (CRI)
    long-tide. *see* long-tide
    mid-tide. *see* fluid tide (mid-tide)
Tiller, William, 59
tissue
    active vs. nonactive interaction with, 17
    biodynamic blueprint guiding, 101–102
    Breath of Life awakening, 73
    CSF carrying potency to, 7
    embryological development and, 132–139, 203
    energetic forces coalescing into form, 6
    experiencing primal midline, 146–147
    fluid tide (mid-tide) and, 78–80, 82
    formative forces and, 2
    inertial fulcrums impacting, 105–108
    inherent treatment plan and, 119–120
    movement of breath and connective tissue, 28
    organizing influence of fulcrums on, 10
    Primary Respiration and, 69–72, 103
    relating to primal midline, 126
    sensitivity to connective tissue (curriculum
        seminar five), 190
    sensitivity to patterns in (curriculum seminar
        three), 189
    shifting orientation from biomechanics to
        deeper forces, 183–184, 186
    Sutherland exploring movements of, 74–75
    Sutherland shifting focus from biomechanics to
        formative forces, 96
    transverse relationships in (curriculum seminar
        seven), 191
    unified field of motion of connective tissue, 7–8
top-down processing, working with trauma, 167–168
torus-shaped bioelectric field
    in embryological development, 132
    form appearing from/in coherent energetic field,
        126–128

touch. *see* physical contact
training programs
    for biodynamic practitioners, 171–172
    in complementary areas, 198–200
    in Continuum and somatic movement
        practices, 204–205
    curriculum, 187
    in embryology, 203–204
    foundation training, 181–182
    online and print resources, 209–212
    options in, 181
    perceptual shift during, 182–187
    postgraduate options, 196–198
    in prenatal and birth psychology and therapy,
        200–203
    prerequisites, 195–196
    for professional registration of practitioners,
        179–180
    requirements (prerequisites), 184
    requirements for, 175
    seminars one through ten in curriculum,
        188–193
    supervision as means of learning and
        supporting, 205–209
transference/countertransference
    curriculum seminar four, 189–190
    impact on relationships, 41–42
    role of supervision, 205
transmutation
    compared with Schauberger's vortices, 130
    generated by Breath of Life, 73
trauma
    awareness in resolution of, 155–159, 173
    coming into present time, 164–168
    Continuum training, 204
    curriculum seminars (two, three, four, and ten),
        188–190, 192
    diagnosing PTSD, 155
    effects of, 154–155
    examples, 152–154
    impact on relationships, 41–42
    issues prompting individual to seek biodynamic
        work, 175–176
    Karuna training programs, 203
    online and print resources, 209–210
    overview of, 149–150
    reactions in therapy sessions related to, 157
    regulating stress response, 191
    resource and, 51, 168–169
    safety and defense and, 159–164
    space, contact, and respect and, 57
    what it is, 150–151
trauma therapy, training programs, 198

triune autonomic nervous system (Porges), 160–164, 191

trust
  establishing/betraying/rebuilding, 54
  impact on relational field, 53–56
  learning to trust, 185–186
  questions to ask potential practitioner, 177–178
  role of trust in settling relational field, 110–113

U

unfolding, inherent treatment plan, 108–110
Upledger, John, 16

V

vagus nerve
  carrying messages between brain and heart, 34
  Polyvagal Theory (Porges), 30
  role in parasympathetic immobilization, 160
  supplying heart and lungs, 32
van der Kolk, Bessel, 199
van der Wal, Jaap, 137, 203
Velasquez, Lizzie, 101, 105
vertebrae/vertebral column
  curriculum seminar five, 190
  notochord and, 135
  potency sensed between L2 and S2, 31
  primal midline running through, 136, 145–146
  spiraling or rising up sensation, 126
vertebrates
  parasympathetic nervous system specializing in immobilization, 160
  role of legs in mobilization, 31
vibration, relating within resonant fields, 58–59
Vipassana meditation, 37, 199
vortices/spirals, energetic organization in nature, 129–132

W

warmth. *see* heat (warmth)
water, resonance and, 59
wave motion. *see also* cranial rhythmic impulse (CRI)
  experiencing primal midline, 147
  exploring CRI settling, 77–78
  exploring long-tide, 85
  exploring mid-tide, 81
  injury presenting as limitation of, 75
  trauma and, 15
webinars, Karuna training programs, 203
websites, 211–212
Western culture
  mind-body split, 173
  orientation to health in, 172
  over-active sympathetic nervous system in Western culture, 27–29
  perceptual shift during biodynamic training and, 185
Winfree, Arthur, 131
Winnicott, Donald
  on allowing clients to rest in being, 26
  on aspects of good-enough holding environment, 56
  concept of relational field and, 53
  on "continuity of being" in undefended state, 46
  on effects of one's relational field, 54
  "good-enough" mothering, 48
Wisdom in the Body (Kern), 73
wounds, role of safety and relationship in healing, 63

Z

"Zero Point Field," 58

ABOUT THE AUTHOR

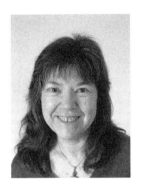

Cherionna Menzam-Sills is certified as a teacher of Craniosacral Biodynamics with the Biodynamic Craniosacral Therapy Association of North America (BCTA/NA) and as a supervisor by the Craniosacral Association of the UK. Authorized as a Continuum Teacher by Continuum founder Emilie Conrad in 2007, Menzam-Sills incorporates this mindful movement practice involving perceptual shifts and healing potential similar to those of Craniosacral Biodynamics into her Biodynamics teaching. With forty years experience teaching and practicing various therapies, mindfulness practices, somatic movement, bodywork, psychotherapy, and prenatal and birth psychology, Menzam-Sills's credentials include degrees in occupational therapy, somatic psychology (dance/movement therapy), and pre- and perinatal psychology, as well as extensive experience with mindfulness meditation and other healing practices. Her doctoral studies led her to develop a uniquely embodied approach to teaching embryology, which she has continued to develop over twenty years, incorporating it into her biodynamic teaching. Her somatic understanding of embryology enhances her sense of universal biodynamic forces guiding our formation both in the womb and in biodynamic session work.

Menzam-Sills teaches Biodynamics and Continuum across North America and Europe, often with her husband, Biodynamics pioneer Franklyn Sills. Before becoming a senior tutor at Karuna Institute, she taught her own biodynamic trainings in Canada and the U.S., as well as guest teaching at the Craniosacral Therapy Educational Trust in London. She has contributed three chapters to Franklyn's pivotal texts, *Foundations in Craniosacral Biodynamics*, volumes one and two, as well as having helped edit them. Through her relationship with Franklyn, Menzam-Sills has accessed new levels of clarity in her understanding and ability to articulate this powerful work. Teaching and discussing Biodynamics with Franklyn have enabled her to embrace an updated, more purely biodynamic approach to craniosacral therapy. She has been immersed in the biodynamic community through being on the Board of Directors of the BCTA/NA and extensive mentoring with Anna Chitty, a senior teacher of Biodynamics in

Boulder, Colorado. She also has presented at biodynamic conferences in the U.S., UK, and Spain, integrating her somatic creativity to engage her audience in the profound mysteries of this beautiful work.

Menzam-Sills lives with Franklyn in an ancient Elizabethan market town in Devon, UK, where she has a private clinical practice that includes supervision with a prenatal and perinatal perspective.

About North Atlantic Books

North Atlantic Books (NAB) is an independent, nonprofit publisher committed to a bold exploration of the relationships between mind, body, spirit, and nature. Founded in 1974, NAB aims to nurture a holistic view of the arts, sciences, humanities, and healing. To make a donation or to learn more about our books, authors, events, and newsletter, please visit www.northatlanticbooks.com.

North Atlantic Books is the publishing arm of the Society for the Study of Native Arts and Sciences, a 501(c)(3) nonprofit educational organization that promotes cross-cultural perspectives linking scientific, social, and artistic fields. To learn how you can support us, please visit our website.